Dear whoever you may be...

This is a 'bookcrossing' book.

I would like you to read whatever you like in it and then pass it on within a month.

My very best wishes to you!

Warm regards,

Lilula

THE SPIRITUAL WISDOM OF INDIA

ABOUT MY SEARCH FOR HAPPINESS
AND THE TRUTH IN LIFE WITH INDIAN
GURUS AND PALM LEAF ASTROLOGERS

VOLUME I

LISBETH EJLERTSEN

authorHOUSE

THE SPIRITUAL WISDOM OF INDIA, Volume 1
- About my search for happiness and the truth in life with
Indian gurus and palm leaf astrologers
© 2017 Lisbeth Ejlertsen. All rights reserved

Danish edition 2017, © FlowLab and Lisbeth Ejlertsen
ISBN 978-87-999608-0-4 (sc)
ISBN 978-87-999608-1-1 (e)
Danish edition 2003, © SphinX Forlag and Lisbeth Ejlertsen
New since 2003: New foreword, new structure, updated chapters, new postscript, new cover

Translation in English by Diane McKennell
Cover photo: Svend Ulsa, Joy Postcards, India
Fonts: Adobe Garamond Pro, Wingdings

Published by AuthorHouse 05/02/2017
ISBN: 978-1-5246-6655-2 (sc)
ISBN: 978-1-5246-6656-9 (hc)
ISBN: 978-1-5246-6654-5 (e)

Web page for this book: www.thespiritualwisdomofindia.com

No part of this book may be reproduced, stored in a retrieval system, or transmitted by any means without the written permission of the author.

Another book in Danish by the same author:
FLOW – FØLG GLÆDEN OG ENERGIEN
Copyright 2007, © Lisbeth Ejlertsen and the publisher Rosinante/GB-forlagene A/S
Copyright 2017, © Lisbeth Ejlertsen and the publisher FlowLab, ISBN 978-87-999608-2-8

Print information available on the last page.
This book is printed on acid-free paper.

Because of the dynamic nature of the Internet, any web addresses or links contained in this book may have changed since publication and may no longer be valid. The views expressed in this work are solely those of the author and do not necessarily reflect the views of the publisher, and the publisher hereby disclaims any responsibility for them.

AuthorHouse™ UK
1663 Liberty Drive
Bloomington, IN 47403 USA
www.authorhouse.co.uk
Phone: 0800.197.4150

CONTENTS

FOREWORD xi

PREFACE BY THE AUTHOR 1
   Facts about the book 1
      Background 1
      The book chose me 1
      2003: 1st publication – in Danish 2
      2017: 2nd publication – in Danish and English 3
      The book follows my journey through 23 years 3
      Target Group 4
      Read all of it or just selected chapters 4
   Preface 1994 – A life-changing journey to India in 1994 5
      My search brought me to India 6
      Who are we as human beings? 6
      What is the meaning of life? 7
      The spiritual roots of India 7
      Gurus and Palm Leaf Astrologers 8
      My starting point 8
      Personal experiences with other dimensions 9
      Open and ready 11
   Preface 1997 – 3 years after the trip 11
   Preface 2001 – 7 years after the trip 12
   Preface 2017 – 23 years after the trip 13
   Volume 2 will be published in autumn 2017 14
   Acknowledgments! 15

DEDICATION 23
To my two Masters 23

THE SPIRITUAL WISDOM OF INDIA 25
Map of India 26

THE SPECIAL QUALITY OF INDIA 27
The allure of India 27
My destinations 27
About searching for happiness 28
The Reunion 29
The Spiritual Face of India 31
Religions versus the Spiritual Philosophy of Life 31

INDIAN SPIRITUAL PHILOSOPHY 35
A simple approach to important concepts … 35
The Vedas – the Oldest Scriptures in the World 36
The Vedas as a Concept 41
The Rishis: the great "seers" of the past 42
The word "OM" or "AUM" – the Universal Sound 42
Sanskrit – The Sacred Language 44
Mantra – Sacred Words 44
The Upanishads – The Spiritual Philosophy of Life 46
The Vedanta Philosophy: everything is oneness 48
The Yoga Philosophy: 8 steps to realisation 49
Kali Yuga: our era 50

HINDUISM 53
The influence of Hinduism throughout the ages 53
The Bhagavadgita – the Hindu "Bible" 54

    The Concept of Bhakti: devotional love 56
    The symbolic language of Hinduism 59
    The Image Symbolism of the Elephant God 61
    The "Infinite Universe" – Brahma, Vishnu and Shiva 66
    Yantra – Geometric Symbols 68

INDIA TODAY – THE LAND OF CONTRASTS 71
    There is something for all the senses 71

A SPECIAL PALM LEAF ASTROLOGER 75
    A little about astrologers and palm leaf astrologers 75
    My first experience with an Indian Palmist 76
    The Meeting with the Special Palm Leaf Astrologer 78
    The Appearance of the Palm Leaves 82
    About the information on my palm leaf 83
    Listen to a little of the recording from the session 89
    How to make use of this 89
    How the Palm Leaves call you 91
    Is Palm Leaf Astrology a Con or a Fact? 92
    Information on prices and places 94

INDIAN GURUS AND MY EXPERIENCES WITH THEM . 101
    What is a guru? 101
    The Task of the True Gurus 102
    My aim in visiting gurus 102
    Ashram: a home for gurus and their students 103
    My attitude to life and "God" 104
    My reactions to the presence of the gurus 105
    A possible explanation for their influence 107
    General remarks about the messages of the four gurus 108
    My experiences with and impressions of each guru 109

    Swamiji 109
    Sai Baba 121
    Amma 124
    Papaji 127
  The addresses of the gurus 135

BACK IN DENMARK 139
  A completely different world 139

POSTSCRIPT 1997 – 3 YEARS AFTER THE TRIP 143
  I meet a new Master and seek clarity 143
  The Master Chariji 145
  My introduction to Sahaj Marg 149
  Transmission – the unique aspect of Sahaj Marg 150
  The Sahaj Marg meditation system in practice 154
  The underlying philosophy of Sahaj Marg 155
  Sahaj Marg's connection with Raja Yoga 156
  Briefly about the cleaning in Sahaj Marg 157
  Definition of "the Self" and "the mind" 159
  Meditation in Sahaj Marg 161
  What is meditation actually? 164
  Why meditation is a necessary instrument 167
  Constant Remembrance – a "Shortcut" 168
  Description of the divine state 174
  Is it necessary to have a spiritual Master? 175
  When is a guru a true Master? 180
  How do you find "Your Master"? 186
  Why only one Master? 187
  Prayer – to whom and for what? 189
  My personal experience with Sahaj Marg 193
  The Seminar in Denmark in 1995 194
  Finding the path to happiness 201
  Sahaj Marg and SRCM – international 204

POSTSCRIPT 2001 – 7 YEARS AFTER THE TRIP 207
- Has the journey in 1994 influence on my life today? 207
- How the palm leaf prophecies worked out 207
  - Would I recommend a palm leaf astrologer? 211
  - Latest news on the special palm leaf astrologer 212
- Newest facts about the gurus I visited in 1994 213
  - Swamiji 213
  - Sai Baba 213
  - Amma 214
  - Papaji 214
- My relationship with Sahaj Marg and Chariji today 215
  - Experiences in Tiruppur, India, 2001 215
- My search for happiness and the truth in life 232
- My goals now and in the future 234

POSTSCRIPT 2017 – 23 YEARS AFTER THE TRIP 237
- Chariji remained my Master 237
- Chariji's successor: Kamlesh D. Patel – Daaji 239
- Heartfulness 242
  - What Heartfulness offers 242
  - Heartfulness Magazine 244
  - Heartfulness – towards the future 246
  - Heartfulness logo 247
  - Further information 248
- New book in autumn 2017: 22 years with the Master 251
- Happiness and the truth in life 253

SOURCES 257
- Sources concerning Indian spiritual philosophy and Hinduism 257
- Sources concerning the four gurus 259
- Sources concerning the postscripts 259
- Sources concerning some illustrations 260

FOREWORD

The quest for Truth or God or Reality in man cannot be traced to any specific period or place. It led man to not only go deeper into the core of his heart, but also to different places in search of a competent Masters who could show the path to realize the Truth hidden in oneself. Thus many people left their homes seeking the guidance of such Masters who usually lived in seclusion, in caves, forests, or mountains, beyond the reach of common man. Millions of others remained content worshipping gods with different names and forms in Temples and other places of worship, often leading to pilgrimage to sacred places.

India is the homeland of spirituality. For several hundred years it has attracted people from different parts of the globe seeking higher knowledge. India is also the land where innumerable texts on varied subjects of Arts, Science, Spirituality, Yoga, Law, Codes of conduct etc. have been written to guide men in the right path. It is said that when Alexander the Great asked his Master Aristoteles before embarking on his long tour to distant lands what he wanted, Aristoteles said: *"If you go to Indika (India) bring a holy man with whom I can discuss things"* [1].

Such is the glory of this holy land that many travellers from Greece, Italy, China, Arabia and other countries have visited this land, travelled length and breadth of this country and documented their appreciation with awe and wonder. Even after numerous invasions by foreigners who

---

[1] *Caturyuga Calendar of Vaivasvata Manvantara (Puranic Chronicles)* by R. Parthasarathy, The Kuppuswami Sastri Research Institute, Chennai, 2015. p.8.

tried to force their ideologies, religious beliefs, customs etc. on to the men of this land, it stands tall without losing its cultural identity, true to the saying that just like all the water falling from the sky reaches the ocean in the form of various rivers, all the prayers addressed to different gods reach but one God.

Vedas are the oldest specimen of literature in this world and they originated in India. Rigveda, the oldest text of this, declares boldly that: *"There is one Reality, but the learned speak of it in different ways"* (Rigveda I.164.46). The Vedic saints had the wisdom and humility to say: *"Let the noble thoughts come to us from all directions"* (Rigveda I.89.1).

In the 19th and 20th centuries great saints like Swami Vivekananda and Rev. Babuji Maharaj (Shri Ram Chandraji of Shahjahanpur, U.P., India), attracted thousands of seekers from all parts of the world. There have been many other religious teachers, preachers and philosophers as well who were adored by thousands of people across the globe.

Lisbeth Ejlertsen of Denmark is one such genuine seeker of Reality. In this book, *The Spiritual Wisdom of India,* she describes vividly her efforts to find solution to the purpose of her life and quench the spiritual thirst. This in turn led her to read a lot of literature pertaining to various religious and spiritual paths.

Her writings on the Vedas in this book, though very brief, are a good introduction to the sacred literature of India and have been presented without any prejudice or bias. She has also given a description of "Nadi" or palm-leaf manuscripts of astrology and how she met both quacks and genuine interpreters of this ancient science of astrology through which the great saints who lived several hundred years ago could predict our present and future.

Lisbeth has also recorded her experiences with four Gurus / Swamijis or spiritual guides of India who have large followers. Her respect for each one is reflected in her writings. Lisbeth's experiences in the Sahaj Marg system of Raja Yoga as practised by the abhyasis of Shri Ram Chandra Mission, a world-wide spiritual organization, her meetings with the great Master Rev. Chariji Maharaj (Shri Parthasarathi Rajagopalachari) and the present Master of the system Rev. Kamaleshji, give us an input of the earnest endeavor of the pining soul to reach its destination.

One can understand from her writings that the seeker should go from "external" to "internal", from "form" to "formless", from "mind" to "heart" and from "unreal" to "real".

This book would stimulate the readers to unravel the mystery of life for which one has to depend on the inner Self, which is possible through the guidance of a worthy Guru.

May this book serve all the people in this direction!

I congratulate Lisbeth Ejlertsen for writing such a wonderful book and wish her to produce more such books for the benefit of humanity!

Chennai, January 3, 2017

Dr. K.S. Balasubramanian

Deputy Director
The KSR Institute,
Mylapore, Chennai – 04.
India

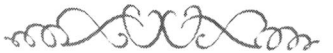

PREFACE BY THE AUTHOR

Facts about the book

This is a book which to me seems magical ... it is as if it has its own agenda and lives a life of its own – as if it controls me and not vice versa ...

Background

During a journey to India in 1994 I had some life-changing experiences. They led me outside the limits with which we in the West define our image of the world. I experienced that it was no coincidence that I found myself in India at precisely that point in time. At the same time I realised that precisely these experiences had been given to me, because I was meant to pass them on to others in our western part of the world.

The book chose me

When I returned to Denmark I wrote three articles during the next few months about my fascinating journey and the spiritual treasures of India. I was satisfied with the result and thus regarded my task as completed. The thought that *I* should write *a book* had never crossed my mind. Nevertheless, the reason that you are sitting with a book and not the three articles is that this book chose me ... That is how I felt right from the start when I realised that the articles had to be put together and expanded into a book if the contents were to go out into the world. In this same, slightly haphazard way, the book has developed through the years. Gradually, the three articles have budded in the course of 22 years into this book with several prefaces and three postscripts. There will also be a sequel to this book which will be published in autumn 2017. It is as if the book itself is in charge of the process.

2003: 1ˢᵗ publication – in Danish

The prefaces and the postscripts were written in the respective years when the book was prepared for publication: 1994, 1997, 2001 and 2017. Not until after the third preparation in 2003 did the book come on to the market in Denmark – nine years after I had written it originally.

It is interesting for me to wonder whether there might be some higher purpose with the nine-year process of publication over which I had no control. Looking back, it seems as if the book had its own agenda. I am well aware that a book is not a living being, but then there must be other powers behind it ...

Although it took a lot of work to compile the articles into a book, I was pleased with the result and relieved to have reached what I thought was the end of the road. I contacted several publishers. First one publisher promised to publish – later another. However, both publishing houses cancelled the agreement when the time for publication drew near. In spite of my frustration at this, I could see with hindsight a purpose with these refusals. On both occasions I had the opportunity to add a new postscript about important steps on my continued path. Among other things, I had met a new teacher whom I found very inspiring. It felt good to be able to introduce him and the method he recommends in the postscript of 1997. In 2001 it made sense that readers could also hear the latest about the steps I have chosen to take later in life.

Therefore, in the big picture, everything was in perfect order in spite of it all.

When the book was finally published in 2003, I felt a great sense of relief that the timing now seemed to be right. The many "ups and downs" throughout the course of things had caused my feelings towards the book to be neutralised. I had let go of all personal expectations and associations with regard to having a book published. I was very glad to place the final full stop when the book was published and let it go completely.

2017: 2nd publication – in Danish and English

Because the book had been out of my universe since 2003, I was very surprised when I received a strong appeal in 2010 to have it translated to English. Some Indian people living in Germany had seen my Danish book. They insisted that Indians living abroad love to gain insight into how foreigners experience them, their culture and their home country – and therefore I *had to* have the book published in English. At the same time as I received this appeal, I could feel a strong energy in my entire body. It set my skin tingling and made me listen ... This feeling of energy is a well-known indicator for me that what is being said is true. Therefore, I interpreted the appeal as an instruction I could not ignore. Obviously, the book wanted to get me out on another journey. The result now in 2017 is that it has yet another postscript. Some updates have been made to the original material where the information was out-of-date or the text was unclear. The book has now been published in both a Danish and an English version and is on sale all over the world.

The book follows my journey through 23 years

The new version of the book covers a period of 23 years during which I have visited India more than 20 times – always searching deeper into the spiritual wisdom of this amazing country. From 1994 to 2017 the book has developed from being about one trip to India to being about my spiritual path of development – my soul's journey through life. It can be said that in the course of these years I started by being curious and inquiring on the surface of the ocean of spirituality, after which I delve deeper down through the years in my quest for the source of everything.

Hearing about an interesting journey is one thing. Following a development through the years and seeing the impact such a journey can have on a person's life is at least as interesting to me. Are the exciting experiences just colourful at the moment of occurrence, after which they fade behind the veil of oblivion? Or do the impressions and the decisions also have an impact in the long run?

My experiences between 2003 and 2017 are numerous. The present book does not have enough room for these. Therefore, a volume 2 will be published in autumn 2017 where I will share more of my special experiences and insights from the latest period.

Target Group

This book is for anyone who is interested in learning more about present day gurus and about Eastern philosophy, culture and spirituality, and especially for those who find it fascinating when factual information is combined with my personal experiences.

Read all of it or just selected chapters

The first three chapters are an introduction to India's spiritual inheritance and culture and cover, among other things, subjects such as the Vedas – the oldest texts in the world, the term Rishis, the universal sound OM, Hinduism, the song Bhagavadgita, god figures with, for example, an animal's head and a human body and the language "Sanskrit" where it is the sound of the words which is important. If you feel a need to find the original context of things and place the concepts in some kind of coherent framework, then it would be a good idea to read the book from the beginning.

If, instead, your primary interest is to gain an insight into my experiences, you can go directly to the chapter: "India today – the land of contrasts".

You can also jump around in the book and read at random. The table of contents is very detailed, so it is easy to spot the chapters that might attract you.

If you wish to know more about the impact a guru has had on my life through 22 years, please be patient until volume 2 is published in autumn 2017.

Preface 1994 – A life-changing journey to India in 1994

Farum, Denmark, autumn 1994

In this book some fascinating experiences are related from a journey in India which I made at the beginning of 1994. Certain things which I witnessed have turned my conceptual universe upside down. When I came home I felt that I was almost under an obligation to pass on my experiences to others who perhaps do not have the means to go there and see things with their own eyes. I think it is important for people to be aware that life holds more possibilities and other dimensions than those with which we are traditionally concerned in our culture here in Denmark and in the entire West. Therefore, it would make me very happy if, by sharing these personal experiences, I can inspire others to find new approaches to their lives and thus discover new possibilities.

My search brought me to India

Searching for happiness and the truth in life is for me the important focal point in my life. It is a lifetime journey. In 1992 I had met a course teacher in Denmark who was very inspired by an Indian Master. I wanted to experience the abilities of the Master for myself. A few months later I visited India for the first time. It was the beginning of a deep connection with this special country to which I knew I would return. Eighteen months later, in 1994, I made the new and life-changing journey to India upon which this book is based.

A specific aim of the trip was to visit various gurus. I wanted to see them with my own eyes materialise objects out of thin air and in this way find certainty that the rumours about these special abilities were true. Another aim was to visit palm leaf astrologers, of whom it is said that they have the whole life course of people written down on palm leaves.

Who are we as human beings?

The desire to go to India sprang from my interest in exploring who we are as human beings and whether there are any limits at all to what we can achieve and accomplish. Old stories about the yogis and gurus of the East indicate that the limits for what is humanly possible are much broader than those which we in the West set for ourselves and our lives. My first trip to India had just whetted my interest in the spiritual side of existence and my desire to search for someone who could do more than what is "normal".

What is the meaning of life?

Spiritual insight gives an idea of what the meaning of life is: that it is the inner, spiritual reality which is the true reality and that the physical world is just an illusion. On the spiritual path you practice "waking" up to the spiritual world via inner contact in the heart. This focus is in sharp contrast to the aims which are most dominant in our western world: material wealth, power and success. For me the Eastern approach to life is fascinating and alluring – a path which I wanted to explore and test to a greater extent.

The spiritual roots of India

To me India seems to be a very special country – in many ways repulsive with its poverty and pollution, but at the same time alluring because of the spiritual foundations of the country and all the spiritual secrets hiding under the surface. As far back in time as is known, the Indian way of life and values have followed the spiritual guidelines and traditions which were written down several thousand years B.C. in the oldest scriptures in the world: the Vedas.

It is an historical fact that there existed Indian sages with a unique insight and knowledge at that time. They "read" nature through their special inner contact with it and documented their experiences and insights in the four Vedas. The knowledge was subsequently assessed by both the sages themselves and the philosophers of the time who were in possession of outstanding analytical abilities. The results became the basis for many sciences, philosophy, astronomy and medicine among others, as well as spirituality, art and several religions, among them Hinduism. Modern research in the West is now only just beginning to arrive at theories and results which are paralleled by knowledge which was intuitively recognised by the sages of those times. Although India's most well-known philosophers lived before our times, their knowledge has not been lost. The gurus and palm leaf astrologers of India are inspired by the spiritual science of the past – interesting people that I wished to visit.

Gurus and Palm Leaf Astrologers

As a Westerner it can be difficult to immediately recognise and appreciate the treasures of India if you know nothing about the country's religious and spiritual background. One will just experience a confusion of temples, gurus and god figures in many colours and shapes. I went there without knowing very much about the religions and the origins of the spiritual view of life. But during the journey my interest in gathering all the various information into a bigger picture was whetted.

In this larger picture the Indian gurus have their natural place as communicators of the spiritual laws and truths. I am talking here about the true gurus ...! Their responsibility is great, and the tasks enormous. They work on the spiritual level for the whole of humanity – never for their own profit's sake. It was important for me to investigate what gurus can do and are already doing for us today.

Palm leaf astrologers are a particularly Indian phenomenon. They pass on a knowledge which has been channelled several thousand years ago to people with insight – a fact which you can choose to reject or investigate further. As I am inquisitive by nature, I was interested in finding out whether there existed an old palm leaf with predictions about my life ...

My starting point

As the form of this book is very personal, because it springs from my interests, opinions, thoughts, feelings and experiences, I find it relevant to give readers an idea of my background and the "glasses" through which I see the world.

The meaning of life, its reasons, mysteries and contexts have interested me greatly for more than 20 years. But in order to be convinced that other people's thoughts and ideas are true and real, I have to experience them for myself. That is why I went to India with precisely that aim in mind: to explore for myself the spiritual wisdom of India. I was 32/33 years old at the time of the trip and had tried my hand at various kinds of jobs: working as an engineer for seven years, a painter for three years and teaching my own courses with the focus on quality of life.

I am a person whose first instinct is to seek a logical and rational explanation for what is happening around me. However, I myself have had experiences which could not immediately be explained in this way. The two most important are described below.

Personal experiences with other dimensions

As a 22 year old newly qualified electronics engineer, I found myself in the middle of a period of depression with only feelings of hopelessness about the future. One day in spring I was standing by the kitchen door in the yard of the house in Copenhagen where I was living. My hand was resting on the door knob and I was about to open the door. All of a sudden there was a clarity in my head – like a ray of sunshine – that took me completely by surprise and did not come from figments of my own imagination. It was as if it arrived inside my head from another dimension. With this clear light I was given to know that everything is transitory. It was not just a logical thought in a normal chain of thought. It was a fundamental certainty which suddenly existed without any connection to what I had been thinking at the time. With this special certainty I understood that being sad would only last for a limited period of time. That this is logically a matter of course is obvious, but even so it is possible to feel that the heaviness and sadness are almost insurmountable just as I was experiencing at that time. But the ray of thought which came to me was different and more than just soothing and consoling words. It contained a truth which was given together with a certainty that this knowledge was a revelation of truth. For many years, with the arrogance of natural science, I had rejected any idea of the existence of anything divine. But this ray of light in my head was so clear and strong that I again became convinced of the existence of something bigger than us human beings in this world. And that this was able to communicate itself to me – in me.

When I was 26, I had another powerful experience in which I was drawn into another dimension than the reality in which I normally exist. The episode took place during a business trip to Turkey. In Istanbul I was standing in front of the Topkapi palace. I was about to walk over and speak to a colleague who was standing about 20 meters away from me. There was a kerbstone on the cobbled pavement. As I went forward, my foot slipped and I lost my balance – a fall could not be avoided. I was annoyed about my accident, but then I wondered why I hadn't fallen yet. The level on which I found myself at that point in time was an unknown place for me. There was absolutely nothing in this space – no connection with my body and no thoughts about it. In the space there were no people, houses or streets – the whole physical world had disappeared. I was completely conscious and could think with my usual feeling that I, myself, was doing the thinking, but the rest of "me" had disappeared. I found myself bathed in a kind of yellowish light, but the light did not have any source. The space was quite empty, but still filled with this light – as if this yellowish light was the "stuff" of which the space of consciousness consisted. My feelings about being in the space were neutral – I was neither afraid nor overwhelmed. My only feeling was a deep sense of wonder at the place in which I found myself. I made an effort to remember what had happened before I suddenly existed in this space. It took a while for me to remember that I had lost my balance and was about to fall. I had no memory of actually hitting the ground. At that moment I realised that I must still be in the process of falling – that is to say in the period of time from when the fall started and before I hit the ground. Such a period of time normally takes fractions of a second, but I experienced it as if several minutes passed in the time pocket in which all this took place. I learned that time is relative and that we, as human beings, have access to several layers of consciousness. At the same moment that I recognised that I was still in the middle of my fall, I was out of this strange sphere of consciousness and back in my body again, after which I immediately hit the ground. Not until then was my fall completed. During the experience I had understood that the human consciousness can exist on several different levels, and that the reality on other levels can appear to be quite different from the physical "reality" which we normally regard as being the only existing reality.

Open and ready

These two experiences of other dimensions have combined to arouse my interest again for the spiritual side of existence. You could say that today I am a mixture of two opposites. My engineering background and rational way of thinking provide a scientific counterbalance to my emotional and intuitive side whose qualities I have learned to listen to and appreciate as the years pass. That is why both my brain and my heart were open and ready for the experiences which I might find in India.

It is my hope that the book will give inspiration to anyone who would like to travel to India, whether on a physical journey or just a journey in mind. India is full of experiences for everyone – those we can comprehend and those that cannot be explained. An Indian Master said about the country:

"India only reveals her beauty for those that love her."

So love her and enjoy her as I do. Bon voyage!

Preface 1997 – 3 years after the trip

Farum, Denmark, spring 1997

About the postscript 1997 – 3 years after the trip:

After the trip in 1994 my interest in exploring the spiritual part of existence continued. The book had not yet been published when I met a new Indian guru in 1995. Parthasarathi Rajagopalachari, also called Chariji. The meeting took place here in Denmark and made a deep impression. It was, therefore, natural for me to also add a postscript about him in the account of my "journey" in search of happiness and the truth in life.

As I still have an urge to achieve a better understanding of the concepts I meet on my quest, this postscript contains a description of the meditation system recommended by Chariji as well as an answer to the important spiritual questions which have arisen on my path. I found clarifying and satisfactory answers with this guru. They gave me the peace of mind to carry out the daily practice which he points to as the shortcut to spiritual goals. Perhaps the answers to these questions might also be interesting to other people – which is why they constitute a large part of this postscript. Among other things, the original meanings are given of the concepts meditation, yoga, the Self, the mind, transmission etc. – as well the reasons given by a Master for his own work.

Preface 2001 – 7 years after the trip

Vrads, Denmark, autumn 2001

About the postscript 2001 – 7 years after the trip:

It is now 2001 – the year I chose to finish this book project. Of course, a lot has happened since my journey in 1994 and also since 1997 when the first postscript was written. Therefore, I have added another postscript to this book which will enable the reader to follow what "the future" has uncovered up until today. I give the status of the predictions I received from a special palm leaf astrologer and tell how my relationship with the four gurus I visited in 1994 has progressed. The postscript also includes news about Master Chariji, whom I chose as my spiritual guide in 1995. The latest information about the gurus and the astrologers has been updated and I answer the question as to whether I have found happiness and the truth in life.

Preface 2017 – 23 years after the trip

Vrads, Denmark, January 2017

About the postscript 2017 – 23 years after the trip:

Everyday life and the spiritual quest are different threads in my existence which through the years have become interwoven to a single fabric. It can no longer be unravelled ... Throughout the years I have experienced that life for us human beings is just different versions of the same themes. I find repeatedly that we humans recognise aspects of ourselves and our experiences in others and their lives. It can be rewarding to share our stories with each other. Therefore, this book still has a very personal angle. I look for this authentic quality of the heart in all of life's situations and among those I associate with. To me this is the most important quality that we as human beings can give each other – to be open, truthful and give each other space to be *whoever we are* with *whatever there is*.

It is with pleasure that I am sending the book out into the world again both in an English and a Danish version. It is now a little more extensive. There are updates here and there and there is a new postscript in which I describe my position in relating to the Master, Chariji, whom I chose as *my* Master. It means a lot to me to show the world both why and how a lengthy and deep relationship with a Master can create value.

However, there is no room in this new postscript for all the exciting and amazing experiences which each in their own way have made me take an extra step towards the Master. They need enough space and, therefore, they will be collected in a new book, a continuation of this one.

We are many who are searching for the spiritual truth. My path is just one of many and precisely the one which calls to me. The thing that makes my path a little different than most people's is the fact that I have sought, found and kept in touch with the same Master through a long period of years. It is this fact – seen from my point of view, which gives my story depth. It would be a pleasure for me if you should find inspiration through this book and that you also feel what is written between the lines ...

Volume 2 will be published in autumn 2017

In the course of the years the book has developed from being about a concrete journey to India to follow the path of my soul. I have moved on from being a seeker among many gurus to following one guide. Whether you call your helper on the path to spiritual development guide, guru, Master or another name, makes no difference. What is interesting is how such a relationship is established and how immersed in it you become.

This book relates how my meeting with my Master arose and also a little about the first stages on my new path together with Him. I am deeply grateful to have experienced that the connection with a true Master can be a lifelong experience. It is my aim to show how very rewarding such a guru can be in a person's life. But as previously mentioned, there is not enough room for many of the important and unique experiences her. They are collected in the sequel – volume 2 – which will be published in autumn 2017. It will be called:

"The Spiritual Wisdom of India, Volume 2" with the subtitle: "22 years with the Master and the path of the Heart – Heartfulness"

My relationship with this book has developed – it is no longer just the book that wants me, I really want it too! In it the deepest part of my heart is reflected – the most valuable thing I have to share. I am very much looking forward to continuing my story in volume 2.

Acknowledgments!

In 1994, when the book was ready in its first version, I expressed my gratitude as follows:

The fact that my material has been transformed into this book has only been possible due to the kind support which I have received in various ways from other people. Therefore I should like to express my HEARTFELT THANKS TO ALL who have contributed during the process. A special thank you to Eric Klitgaard, who with his professional approach gave the first proposal for the book's outer appearance so that it matched my vision, to Jens Gnaur who, with his great knowledge of Indian philosophy of life and history, has guided me to a greater understanding of this field, and to Jens Clausen and Jytte Gravesen who, by sharing their insight and many years of experience in Sahaj Marg meditation, have increased my clarity and openness to what cannot be described.

Here in 2017 I would like to extend this thank you to also include many others:

Through the years I have learned that some initiatives unfold in strange ways, while other things which I have struggled to achieve were not able to thrive and grow. Today I am convinced that there is a greater meaning with everything that happens in our lives as human beings. We are all given help to unfold the plan for our lives – the plan laid by our soul before we were born. I have a sense that energy beings from other worlds help us as much as they may and can. My heartfelt thanks go, therefore, also to all helpers without name or form who guide us unseen on the path which our soul has chosen to follow in this life. Thank you for whispering in my ears and those of others with the result, among other things, that we have been open to this book project!

At the same time, my heartfelt thanks to the people who have listened to this whisper and given their crucial contributions to the new version of the book.

- Indian Jayakumar Ramamurti and his wife Gowri Sankaran: Thank you both for inspiring me to have the book translated and repeatedly insisting on this until I got the work done!
- My mother, Else Ejlertsen: Thank you for listening to the thought which was sent to you about giving an inheritance advancement to your three daughters. This financial helping hand created the opening for the translation to get started! Thank you for all your love and your unlimited support for my projects even when others could not see the point of them ...!
- Language advisors Tina Korup and Karin Sode: Thank you for your persevering support in finding the right translator, so that the English version came to match the Danish one ...!
- Translator Diane McKennell: Thank you for superbly bringing the spirit of the book into the English version – and thank you for being willing and able to take on a task on untraditional

conditions! Your patience with my delays has been a great support and gift!
- Bjørn Drengsgaard, methodical man of many talents: Thank you for in many ways being the facilitator for the new version, keeping track of details and making sure that the new Danish version appears in correct Danish – your contribution gives me a sense of safety ...!
- To Dr. Kannan S. Balasubramanian, a scholar of Sanskrit and the deputy director of the Kuppuswamy Shastri Reasearch Institute in Chennai, India: Thank you so much for taking the time to write the foreword for this book and also for checking my writings about the Indian Spiritual Philosophy. You are a very inspiring person to listen to and spend time with – it has been a pleasure to meet you!
- Members of the Heartfulness Institute:
  Elizabeth Denley: Thank you for your advice and for making sure that all the information about Heartfulness is correct – and thanks for your inspiration for the cover of volume 2 in India and for your amazing help in getting things to happen, Ravi Chaudhary: Thank you for your quick and professional help to obtain all QR codes Rishabh C. Kothari: Thank you for your guiding vision and care that choices were made in accordance with the Master's wishes.
- Photographer Sven Ulsa: Thank you very much for letting me borrow your fantastic postcard for the cover of this book and volume two coming out next year. And fantastic that your trusted me enough to lend me the original picture – the only link you had to the postcard. It says a lot about your heart ...!
- Graphic designer Susan Bach Andersen: Thank you for meeting me with heartfelt openness and a wish to help me with the graphic design – your promises can always be trusted!
- My lovely artist-daughter, Signe Emine Petersen: Thank you very much for wanting to contribute with the drawings I needed – you are an angel and an invaluable gift to my life!

- Photo enthusiast Gunver Mossin Kofoed: Thank you for being ready for both types of cover photo – I enjoy the positive time we spend together.
- Photographer Mona Srinivas Bandaru: Thank you for taking the time to take photographs in India for the cover of volume 2 and at the same time allowing me to enjoy your presence and warmth.
- Illustrator and artist Nanna Ernst: Thank you for your beautiful drawing of Amma which captures both her warmth and fantastic radiance – and thank you for transforming the picture of me to such a fine drawing which symbolises the simplicity on the spiritual path.
- The originators of the publishing house AuthorHouse: Thank you for founding this publishing house whose aim it is to help people like me to bring out into the world the material that means so much to us! It was only due to the fact that I discovered this easy shortcut to the foreign book market that I found the courage to launch the project with an English version of my Danish book.
- A big thank you also to all the capable employees at AuthorHouse, especially Donald Stephans: So good, Donald, that you persuaded me to publish volume 1 the year before volume 2 – it has given space and free energy, and thank you for your support in getting the whole process of publication back on track.
- Concerning all other photos and drawings which have been lent to me under the condition that they are all the intellectual property of those organisations and that all rights are reserved: I would like to thank you from the bottom of my heart for having been so accommodating to me!

Thank you for all photographs relating to Sahaj Marg and Heartfulness which have been reprinted here with permission from Shri Ram Chandra Mission and Heartfulness Institute, Thank you to Mr. Shyam Pai for permission to reprint the drawing of the Hindu god, Dattatreya, from the cover of the book Sadguru Dattatreya which was written and published by his father, Sadguru Sant Keshavadas from Bangalore, India, and also a big thank you to Mr. Abhishek Jain, Motilal Banarsidass Publishers (P) Ltd. in India and to Mr. Ashok Jain, Munshiram Manoharlal Publishers Pvt. Ltd. in India for your great help in finding the author's family,

Thank you to author Mr. A. Parthasarathy at VedantaWorld in India for the drawing of Ganesha,

Thank you to the palmist Mr. A. Sivasamy for lending me private photos of palm leaves,

Thank you to Mr. Prasad, Swamiji's ashram, for lending me the photo of Swamiji and the illustration of the symbol Sri Chakra,

Thank you to my wonderful and helpful friend, Louis Jeppsson, for establishing the contact to Mr. Prasad,

Thank you to Amma-Danmark, Lilian Bjerregaard og Nanna Aakard for your persistent efforts in trying to obtain permission to reproduce the photo of Amma,

Thank you to Sri Sathya Sai Sadhana Trust, Publications Division for lending me photos of Sai Baba,

Thank you to Sri Ramana Marhashi's Ashram, Sri Ramanasramam in India for lending me photos of Ramana Maharshi,

Thank you to Lennart Nordstrand for private photos and to Eric Klitgaard for photos of our Master.

- Concerning the permissions to reproduce the contact information given in the book:

Thank you to palm leaf astrologer, Mr. A. Sivasamy, for contacts concerning the palm leaf office,

Thank you to Swamiji's Ashram Office in Mysore for contacts concerning Swamiji,

Thank you to Sri Sathya Sai Sadhana Trust, Publications Division for contacts concerning Sai Baba,

Thank you to Amma Media Team for contacts concerning Amma,

Thank you to Vandita, Papaji's Satsang Bhavan, for contacts concerning Papaji and
Thank you to the Heartfulness Institute for contacts concerning Heartfulness.

- Last but not least – thanks to everyone – gurus and ordinary people who have accepted me on my travels and each given their contribution to my adventure!

DEDICATION

To my two Masters ...

I dedicate this book to my two spiritual Masters – a greeting from my heart which is filled with love and gratitude:

Parthasarathi Rajagopalachari, Chariji

THANK YOU for calling me to you without words. You were the foundation for my spiritual inspiration and development throughout the 19 years I have known you and we were able to meet in the physical world. Through countless experiences, both in your physical proximity and also when you were somewhere else in the world, you gave me, directly and indirectly, the material for this book and its sequel – volume 2. I look forward to taking all my future steps inspired by you from the spiritual world. I am eternally grateful for everything you have given me.

Kamlesh D. Patel, Daaji

THANK YOU for accepting the task of Chariji's successor. No one except the Masters themselves know the deprivation and responsibility involved in this task. To the world and to me it is the greatest gift that you are there like a lighthouse showing how to chart the course so as to arrive at the right harbour. I know it is only possible to catch glimpses of the help you give to us all. Thank you for your support in big and small things – also for this book project.

THE SPIRITUAL WISDOM OF INDIA

ABOUT MY SEARCH FOR HAPPINESS
AND THE TRUTH IN LIFE WITH INDIAN
GURUS AND PALM LEAF ASTROLOGERS

Map of India

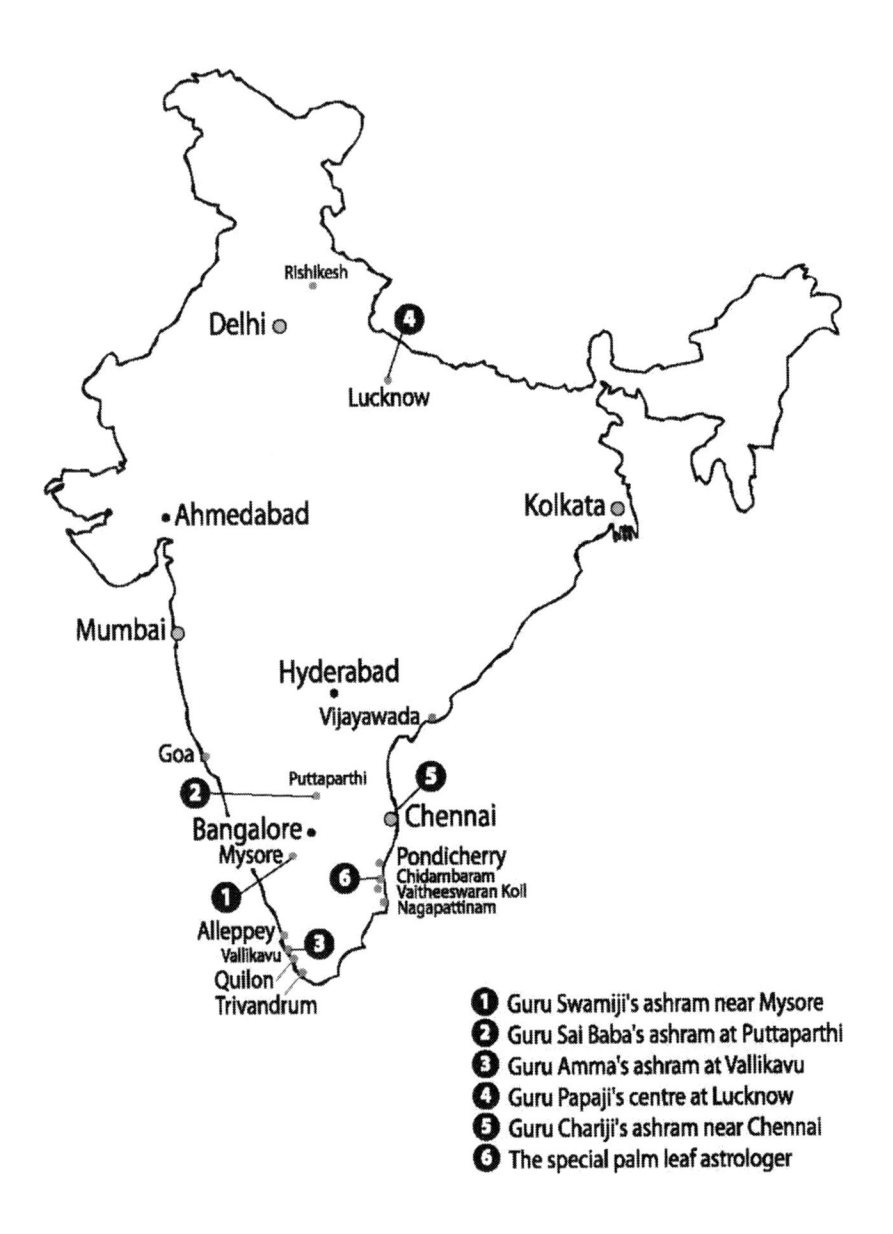

❶ Guru Swamiji's ashram near Mysore
❷ Guru Sai Baba's ashram at Puttaparthi
❸ Guru Amma's ashram at Vallikavu
❹ Guru Papaji's centre at Lucknow
❺ Guru Chariji's ashram near Chennai
❻ The special palm leaf astrologer

Drawing: Susan Bach Andersen

THE SPECIAL QUALITY OF INDIA

The allure of India

Is it really necessary to go all the way to India AGAIN? That was the not unexpected reaction of my family to my decision to leave the safety of Denmark once again. My aim was another journey to the other side of the globe. Eighteen months earlier I had defied my love of comfort and fear of the unknown by going there to visit the Indian Master Poonjaji. The experience had reinforced my desire for adventure. The atmosphere, energy and nectar for the heart which I had caught the scent of was enticing me and could not be conjured away. I wanted to search for more of the wisdom to be found in this land full of contrasts. I had no choice, I had to go back.

My destinations

My plan was to visit the four gurus Ganapati Sachchidananda Swamiji, Sathya Sai Baba, Mata Amritanandamayi and H.W.L. Poonjaji. The map in Figure 1 shows where the four gurus have their home bases and that these addresses are spread around the country. For me the journey was not about finding a personal guru to bind my life to in the future. But meeting Poonjaji had whetted my appetite for visiting other similar characters in order to experience their various facets of divine wisdom.

Palm leaf astrologers are a particularly Indian phenomenon. It is said that the astrologers can tell you everything about the past and present of those people whose life history was written down on palm leaves more than 3,000 years ago. It sounded incredible to my ears, but also fascinating and worth investigating. When I decided to look for these people, I had no data or addresses to start with, but had only made this aim clear in my mind.

About searching for happiness

If the truth must be told, I have to admit that the underlying purpose of the whole journey was of course a quest for happiness. Since I was 16 it had been my firm decision to live a life in which I felt happy. But what is happiness precisely? Is it a state? Or is it a thing? The aims and ways which our Western ideals point to in the form of power, riches and "having the right look" all seem to come to a dead end. Now and again I have had a glimpse of the state of happiness at the gateway of a goal, but after a while the frustration always returns, because this state of happiness does not last for ever. This dissatisfaction sows the seeds of a new desire which then becomes the new goal in the endless quest for eternal happiness. The state of happiness cannot be identified with "the thing" which seems to have triggered it. After a while, the happy buyer of a new house can be just as happy to get rid of the house again. So it is not the house itself which constitutes the happiness. If "the thing" cannot sustain the state of happiness, does that then mean that our state of happiness is only determined by how we *relate* to the things – and to life?

How to stop hunting for things and how to experience the state of happiness in the Now is the cardinal point in Eastern philosophy. This means trying to let go of every desire and wanting something other than what is already there. The spiritual Masters say that the state of happiness is always within us. When we remove our gaze from the fruits of desire to the Now and let it rest there, then we will encounter it. Although these ideas come from a culture whose origins are several thousand years old, being a human being has not changed much. Physically we have the same limbs and on the mental level the same resources and channels. I find the ideas of the Masters fascinating and alluring, but find it difficult to live in accordance with them in practice. Perhaps new inspiration from palm leaf astrologers, gurus or from the Indian culture will make a difference ...

The Reunion

So there I was suddenly, in the heat and the dusty, polluted air, in the midst of the chaotic rush hour traffic, as only it can be in India. I was on the road between the airport and the station in the large Mid-Indian town of Hyderabad heading towards Vijayawada. It was in the vicinity of this town that the guru Swamiji was to be found at that time. Back home I had learned that he was going on tour and that my chance to meet him would be to seek him out in this place during the next four days. Revisiting everyday Indian life was pure joy, although I both loved and hated this reality. The absolutely most predominant drawback was the bluish-black reek of the traffic lying like a blanket over most of the Indian towns. It is impossible to breathe freely with everything smelling of soot, dust and smoke. So I was rather surprised that I was now sitting in a scooter-rickshaw just enjoying my renewed encounter with India. Perhaps it is the Indian mentality which overshadows all the drawbacks. The traffic is completely chaotic, but glides along all the same. There is room for even the meanest bicycle-rickshaw on the overcrowded roads where the traffic is completely without structure and rules. Cars and other vehicles are all just about falling apart. In a country where the inhabitants only learn to move about in traffic by being in it, the laws of nature apply: the biggest road

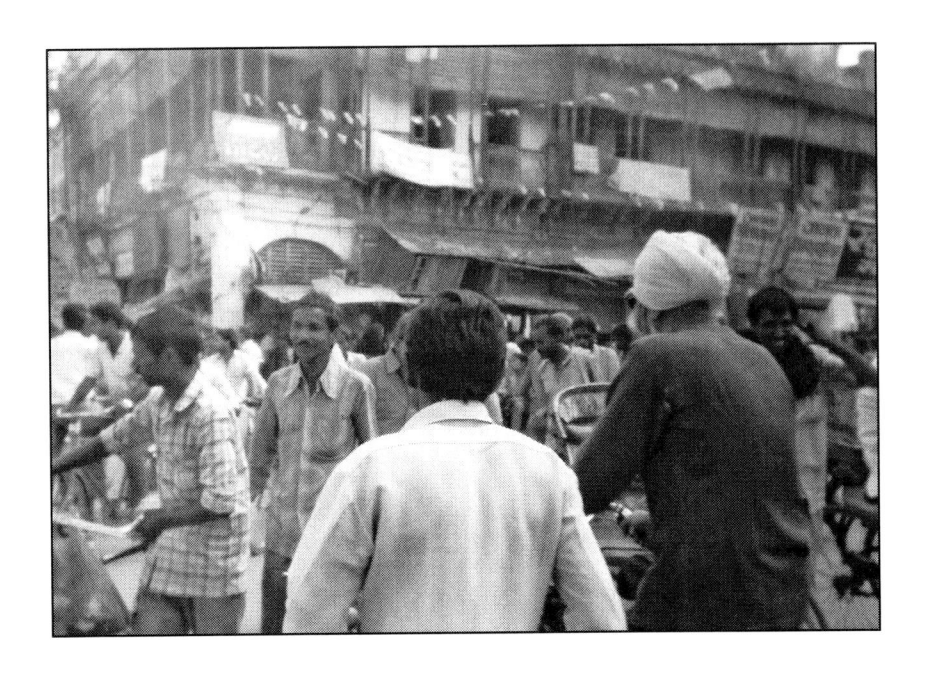

A street scene from the bazaar district in Lucknow. Photo: Lisbeth Ejlertsen

users call the shots. Even so, the motorists make allowances for the cyclists, because the latter may not realise how vulnerable they actually are. Even the pedestrians move along through the traffic at their own kind of sleep-walking pace, the cars just drive round them. The few Indians I have seen running were beggars pursuing their victims. In this Indian inferno there is only one thing to do: find your own inner calm and let yourself be whirled along by the current. That was how I found myself in the midst of this joy of revisiting India.

This calm, which had replaced my excitement and frustration during the plane trip coming here, was to become a good travelling companion during the whole trip. When I finally gave way to the stress and tears on the way to Mumbai, all that was left were calm and warmth. Now the pressure and worries in Denmark before my departure were left behind. I was happy and contented that I had taken the plunge again into a new adventure.

The Spiritual Face of India

India is a country where people with great spiritual insight have lived throughout the ages. Or else it is just the country where these such people have been allowed to become known, because their work was supported by the people. You see, searching for *the truth in life* is an essential part of Indian culture and tradition. For Indians, yoga comes before football. They love and worship their gurus and yogis as teachers that can lead them to their goal: to become at one with the divine. The yogis prove that by means of physical exercises and concentration it is possible to master the bodily functions way beyond the limits which we in the West believe to be possible. It has been scientifically proven that some of these yogis are able to hold their breath for several hours, make their hearts stop and consume lethal poisons without these extreme influences changing their physical well-being. These phenomena show that their view on humanity holds possibilities that we in the West do not believe exist. In India the concept of God is still alive in the people today. Aspiring to spiritual values and development is an essential part of the everyday life and aim in life for many Indians.

Religions versus the Spiritual Philosophy of Life

The basic difference between the view of religions on the relationship between God and humans and the spiritual philosophy of life is that religions define God as being outside humans and view humans as basically sinful. Conversely, the spiritual philosophy of life assumes humans to be divine beings, because God is a concept which is omnipresent at all times and, therefore, also the substance of which we humans consist.

In religions where God is outside humans there is room for a priesthood which can undertake the role of intermediary between God and humans. Because God is so abstract, the priests can almost set the agenda themselves as to how people should behave and what they must do to obtain absolution and get their "ticket" to everlasting life in Paradise. If you look at the riches owned by the churches/priests in the various religious persuasions, you could easily suspect these "intermediaries" of feathering their own nests. Also many wars have been fought in the name of God, perhaps in reality as a cover for humans' own lust for power.

In contrast, the basic idea in the spiritual philosophy of life is that in order to meet God or the Divine Essence we must search for it in our own hearts. There is no external definition of this Divine Essence, because it cannot be described. But it can be experienced, and humans experience with their hearts and not with their heads. In this context the purpose of life is to establish contact with this essence and live life on the basis of that being.

INDIAN SPIRITUAL PHILOSOPHY

A simple approach to important concepts ...

Throughout time the innermost nature and essence of being has been viewed from various angles by the Indian spiritual philosophy. The changing cultural, political and religious currents have naturally influenced the way in which we relate to spiritual life. Even so, it is characteristic for precisely this country that there are a certain number of religious and spiritual scriptures which have had and continue to have a quite decisive influence. The oldest and most well-known works are: The Vedas, the supplementary Vedic literature, among others the Upanishads, as well the epic poem Bhagavadgita. It is mainly the ideas from these that have formed the basis of the Indian view of life and the world throughout the past 3-4,000 years. At that time the people were analytically and scientifically oriented. They wished to systematise and understand things correctly. The thoughts and ideas of the past on the origin and purpose of life are also relevant and interesting today. Both in the Hindu religion and in the messages from many of the present day spiritual gurus, reference is constantly made to these old scriptures which form the basis of religions as well as the spiritual view of life.

So when an ignorant Dane begins to take an interest in the Indian philosophy of life, it is a bit like trying to find your way through a maze. You soon meet the word "Veda", but it is used both about actual scriptures and as a concept – this can give rise to some confusion. Other words such as "OM" or "AUM", "Sanskrit", "Vedanta", "Yoga" and "Rishi" occur again and again, and reference is made to the Bhagavadgita. These words and concepts are all essential for understanding Indian spiritual philosophy; so they are explained as briefly and simply as possible in this and the next chapter.

The Vedas – the Oldest Scriptures in the World

The Vedas are not only the oldest scriptures in India, but the oldest in the whole world. The Vedas consist of four collections. Some people believe that they originate from way back about the year 4,000 BC, while others date them to about the year 1,500 BC. (see sources 4, 6, 7 and 13). It is difficult to know the precise date for several reasons, one of which is the fact that stories at that time were traditionally handed down by word of mouth. The Vedas may have existed for several hundred years in this form before being written down. Moreover, the writing process itself took place over a longer period of time. And finally, the Indians of that time regarded time as mystical and were, therefore, not interested in dating the scriptures themselves. In order to date the origins of the Vedas it has been necessary to rely on indications in the texts and compare them with archaeological finds.

The word "veda" itself means "knowledge". The knowledge described by the Vedas concerns the very substance of the universe, its laws and contexts. The four Vedas, which are partly written in verse and partly in prose, are called Rigveda, Sāmaveda, Yajurveda and Atharvaveda. The oldest of these is the Rigveda. This conclusion is partly based on the fact that large parts of it are repeated or are assumed to be known in the three others (see source 4 p. 842). The Atharvaveda is the most recent. Rigveda is also called Rgveda. In source 4 page 649 this oldest source dates from between 2,500-2,000 BC – i.e. it is about 4,000 years old.

The fact that the Vedas were created over a long period of time is expressed in their different types of content. The Rigveda reflects in a simple and beautiful manner on how a people, whose development had come beyond the basic demands of nature, related to the forces of nature. The other three Vedas show signs of the existence of a strong, established priesthood in their time. These texts contain many formulas and instructions which only the priests may use in their ritual work. In broad outline the contents of each individual Veda can be summarised as follows:

Rigveda: the name means "hymns",
it contains for the most part hymns based on worldly life praising various gods. However, it also has a smaller part which is more spiritually orientated concerning the "Universe" – the abstract, unlimited and vague god concept,
it consists of 10 books containing 1,017 hymns with 10,472 verses in all (see source 4 pp. 649 and 842)

The Sāmaveda: the name means "the song veda",
melodies and songs with instructions for the work of the priests, in particular the sacrifices,
it consists of 400 hymns with 1,549 verses (see source 13 p. 200)

The Yajurveda: the name means "offer veda",
handbook with rituals and mantras (prayers) for the sacrifices of the priests, the purpose of which was to have various types of wishes fulfilled.

Yajurveda has been recorded and written down via two different processes and channels, each of which has created its own school: the "White School" and the "Black School", respectively. The "White School" is also called "Sukla". The texts in the White School are better organised and concern prayers for the more positive aspects. The "Black School" is also called "Krishna". The texts in the Black School are more disorganized and contain descriptions of many rituals and sacrifices, the White School, which consists of 40 books, has over 2,000 verses, the Black School consists of 7 khāndas [chapters] (see source 4 pp. 842 and 892 and source 5)

The Atharvaveda: the name Atharva is another name for God, magic formulas and incantations, among others, for undoing any mistakes made during the priests' sacrifices and to heal sickness and help restore the harmony of the body, and to have wishes fulfilled and attain prosperity in several areas of life, for exorcising evil spirits and celebrating the omniscience and power of God, it consists of 20 books containing more than 700 hymns with approx. 6,000 verses in all (see source 4 pp. 72 and 842 and source 13 page 33)

One of the sciences which originate from the teaching of the Vedas is āyurveda. This traditional treatment of illness in India is based on the guidelines about body and mind presented by the Arharvaveda. The word "āyurveda" means "the truth about life". Today this treatment is also available in the West.

Among the four scripture collections – the Vedas – the Rigveda is not only the oldest, but also the most beautiful and easiest to comprehend. As previously mentioned it consists of poems about and to the gods of nature and is written by poets and thinkers. The texts express wonder at the whole mystery of creation and they relate to life, death and ethical issues. But it is not an unequivocal view of the universe and the divine origin which is expressed in the Rigveda. The starting point in most of the texts is that there are many gods and that the forces of nature are each subjected to their own god. For example, the god of fire Agni, the storm gods Maruts, the sun god Surya and the god of thunder is called Indra. The latter is also the king of the gods. Sacrifices and incantations were used to try to influence the conditions of life towards what they hoped to achieve or away from what they wished to avoid. And yet in a few of the Rigveda's texts you will find the spiritual idea that there is only one divine source and that you must search for it via your own heart. The following two quotations illustrate these two completely different views of the divine origin:

The first example from the Rigveda (10.16) is an excerpt from a burial hymn. It is addressed to the god of fire Agni to ask for the best possible help for the deceased's onward journey. First Agni is asked to prepare the body in the best possible way and then to pass it on to his forefathers. They and the will of the gods will lead the deceased to his right home from where the person originated. The hymn testifies that body and spirit are not considered as two completely different elements:

"Do not burn him entirely, Agni, or engulf him in your flames. Do not consume his skin or his flesh. When you have cooked him perfectly, O knower of creatures, only then send him forth to the fathers.

When you cook him perfectly, O knower of creatures, then give him over to the fathers. When he goes on the path that leads away the breathe of life, then he will be led by the will of the gods.

[To the dead man:]) *May your eye go to the sun, your life's breath to the wind. Go to the sky or to earth, as is your nature; or go to the waters, if that is your fate. Take root int the plants with your limbs."* [Later in the hymn sacrificial gifts are brought to Agni.] (see source 3 p. 49 verse 1-3)

The other example from the Rigveda (10.129) is an excerpt from a creation hymn in which the spiritual view of life is expressed:

"... The life force that was covered with emptiness, that one arose through the power of heat.

Desire came upon that one in the beginning; that was the first seed of mind. Poets seeking in their heart with wisdom found the bond of existence in non-existence." (see source 3 p. 25 vers 3-4)

However, as previously mentioned, temporal life and material goods rather than spiritual interest are the predominant features of the Rigveda. The aim of most of the texts was to influence the forces of nature in particularly critical situations. There were ceremonies for events such as birth, death and marriage as well as social changes such as the appointment of a new king. The Rigveda also contains prayers and incantations for everyday situations which could be difficult to manage, for example becoming pregnant, dealing with rivalry and achieving beauty.

The fact that the Vedas consist of rules, rituals and other help for living in accordance with the gods and the spiritual truth gives a picture of how important the divine aspect was and is to the Indian people. The Vedas represent the very backbone of all Indian spiritual philosophy.

The Vedas as a Concept

It can be difficult to form a clear picture of what the Vedas actually are. Because the word "Vedas" is used both in connection with the four books previously mentioned and sometimes also as a designation for the four books together with the supplementary Vedic literature which consists of philosophical reflections on the four books. Last but not least, the word "Veda" is used as a concept.

The concept of Veda comprises the entire universal knowledge about the very mystery of nature. In this connection, Veda is a *universal state* in which this all-encompassing knowledge is revealed. Thus the contexts in nature are always present and accessible to anyone who has achieved the necessary spiritual state. Highly developed people such as these will automatically *experience* the Vedas which will reveal themselves to them. Hence the concept of Veda is not concerned with philosophical ideas conceived by the human brain. Instead the Vedas in this context are a blueprint – an impression – of the universe. The people who view reality from this approach believe that the universe was created by a sound, and that it is this sound itself which is the creating force (see source 4 p. 843). Because this knowledge of the sound of creation and the laws of nature are always omnipresent, the Vedas as a concept have no beginning and no end. They describe everything that has been, is and will be.

Therefore the concept of Veda is not identical with the four collections of scriptures. Many people believe that the pronunciation itself – that is the sound – of the Veda scriptures is a reflection of the universal Veda state. Thus the texts become divine revelations – a point of departure which is not questioned. Seen in this context, it is extremely vital that the prayers and incantations of the Veda scriptures are recited absolutely correctly, because the sounds themselves are the creating force. With the right sounds a person wishes to waken the forces in nature which can fulfil his or her desires. In source 33 the Veda concept is explained as follows:

"Veda is really that condition which was before the time of the creation of the universe ... Therefore it is quite true that the Vedas came in to exixtence at the time of the creation of the universe. They have been shaped into the form of books. It is as if the conditions have been given a dress." (see source 33 p. 323)

Many present day Indians regard the Vedas as divine revelations.

The Rishis: the great "seers" of the past

"The authors" of the Veda scriptures are called Rishis. The word "rishi" means "seer". The designation reflects the view that these Rishis were in possession of such a high level of consciousness that they directly saw and experienced the spiritual truths and hence the Veda scriptures are a reproduction of this insight. There have existed many of these Rishis in India and they come from all castes and levels of society. The number of Rishis throughout the times is approximately 48,000 (see source 4 p. 651).

The word "OM" or "AUM" – the Universal Sound

The word "OM" is an obvious example of the Veda concept. To Indians this word, which is pronounced AUM, is the symbol for *the whole universe*. Because when AUM is correctly pronounced, all sounds are contained in just this one word. It is believed that AUM is the very

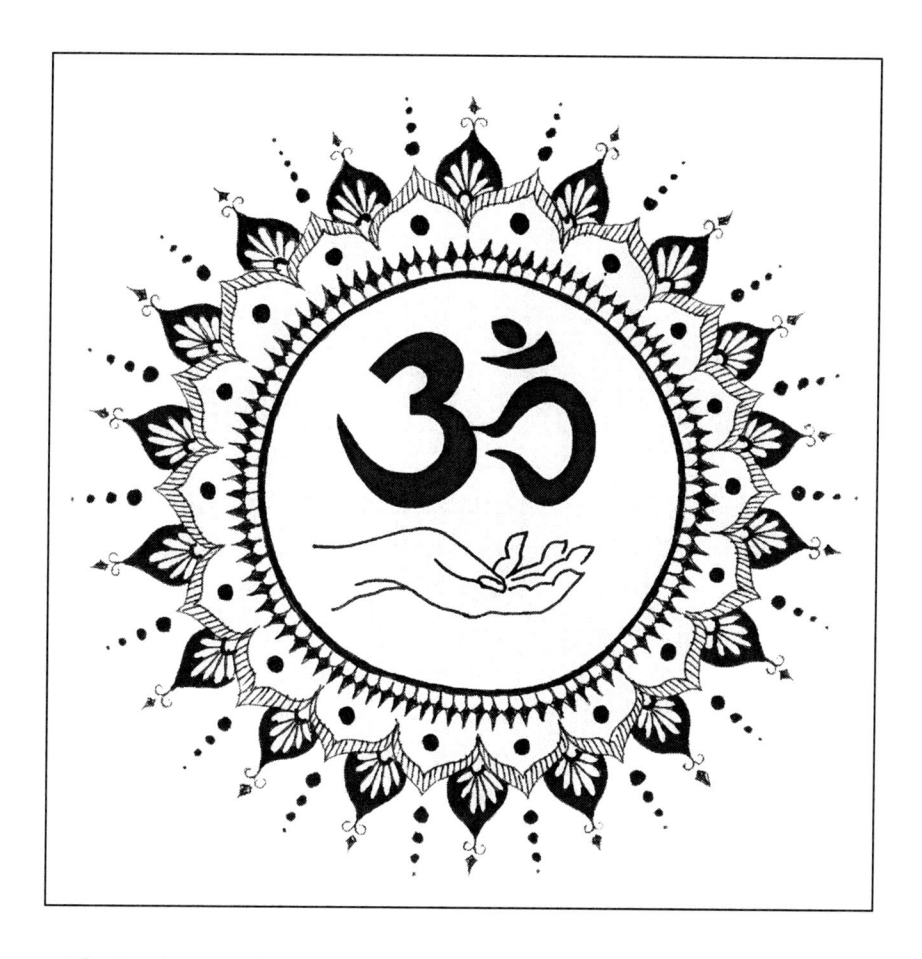

The Sanskrit sign for the sound OM/AUM. Drawing: Signe Emine Petersen

sound with which the universe was created. The correct pronunciation of the word starts at the back of the throat with A. This sound is allowed to rise up through the throat while simultaneously changing to a U. On its way from the throat around the mouth towards the lips the U sound becomes an M. The sound finishes right at the front at the tip of the lips. In this way the pronunciation of AUM goes through the whole human sound range – all sounds have been pronounced (see source 16 p. 127).

The three letters of the primeval sound, A, U and M, also symbolise everything else in the universe. For every thing or movement has a beginning (like the beginning of the primeval sound's beginning: A), it is maintained for a while (like the middle part of the primeval sound: U) and it has an ending (like the ending of the primeval sound: M) (see source 10 p. 24-38). Therefore the word "AUM" is considered to be an expression for the universe and consequently for God.

Sanskrit – The Sacred Language

The concept of Veda is also expressed in the Sanskrit language. It is an old and sacred Indian language from the time of the Vedas. The reason for referring to it as sacred is that it is the human reproduction of the universal sounds which were detected at that time. The graphic characters were created by reproducing the form of the sound vibrations which were felt. The language was named "Sanskrit", because this word means "divine" (see source 33 p. 311). The Indian Master, Babuji also writes as follows about the alphabet in this language:

"If you deeply ponder over the alphabet of Sanskrit you shall find the rise and fall in it in the form of natural vibration. And in that language, they have written by feeling every vibration: and they started to call it Sanskrit (Divine)." (see source 33 p. 327)

Mantra – Sacred Words

It is known that the sound of special words triggers certain impacts in the universe. This knowledge, which was experienced by the Rishis, inspired human beings to exert influence on the energies of the universe themselves by means of sound. By using special words or sentences, attempts are made to activate the universal energies which support and fulfil one's own intents and purposes. These individual words or combinations of words are called mantras. A mantra is a kind of prayer, except that you do not pray to a god, but set things in motion yourself. Therefore, a mantra can be called a kind of magic formula.

For example, the word "AUM" is used as a mantra when you want to come into contact with the universal entity. Other mantras can be much more worldly in character, such as the hymns from the Vedas which were used to achieve fertility.

A common factor for the mantras is that they consist of words in Sanskrit. One of the oldest and most well-known mantras which is used to achieve spiritual development is called Gayatri. It was originally mentioned in the Rigveda and consists of 24 words meaning:

"We meditate on the glory of that Being who has produced this universe; may He enlighten our minds." (see source 24 p. 13)

In Sanskrit the text of the mantra is this:

*"Om Bhur Bhuva Suvah
Tat Savitur Varenyam
Bhargo Devasya Dheemahi
Dhiyo yo nah prachodayat"*
(see source 16 p. 134)

Some people repeat this mantra both at sunrise and sunset. The mantra is repeated 108 times by some practitioners at these points in time. Both the person saying or singing the Gayatri mantra and the person listening to it are cleansed by it. It is said of this mantra that this sacred prayer spreads out in a spiral form throughout the whole universe from the heart of the person singing it with an appeal for peace and divine wisdom for everyone. This is why this mantra is used by some people as an impersonal universal prayer for the world.

The Upanishads – The Spiritual Philosophy of Life

The slightly mystical and divine character of the Vedas and their – at times – implied and abstract texts have given rise to many philosophical reflections. They occur as comments, interpretations and other supplementary literature. The supplementary scriptures, which are directed at different groups of seekers of the divine, can be divided into the following four categories (see source 4 p. 808):

Samhitās,	which, among other things, are hymns praising the gods,
Brāhmanas,	with instructions for the prayers and ceremonies of the priests,
Āranyakas,	which are directed at hermits in the forests and
Upanishads,	which are reflections of a more philosophical nature.

The Vedas themselves contain over one million verses, while the supplementary Vedic literature is so comprehensive that it is not possible to read all of it in the course of a lifetime.

It is in the Upanishads that the spiritual philosophy of life is expressed in earnest. The word "upanishad" means "sitting at the feet of the Master". At that time people gathered there to receive his wisdom. The texts in the Upanishads reflect an unprejudiced wonder at life as well as sincerity and tolerance. The thoughts which are expressed have been the seed of many philosophical systems and schools of thought. Although these systems all originate from the same source, they indicate different roads to becoming a perfect human being. *Yoga* and *Vedanta* are the names of two of the most widespread philosophical systems from the Upanishads. They are described in more detail in the following subsections.

The meaning of the universal sound OM/AUM and the path to attaining the divine state is also described in several places in the Upanishads. The first of the two following quotations comes from the Maitri Upanishad. In this text the name Brahman is a designation for the impersonal universe – identified by the sound OM. The goal lies beyond this where you will find an omnipresent silence of joy. This goal is identified here with Vishnu. The word "contemplation" means inner absorption in the self.

"The sound of Brahman is OM. At the end of OM there is silence. It is a silence of joy. It is the end of the journey where fear and sorrow are no more: steady, motionless, never-falling, ever-lasting, immortal. It is called the omni-present Vishnu. In order to reach the Highest, consider in adoration the sound and the silence of Brahman. For it has been said: God is sound and silence. His name is OM. Attain therefore comtemplation – contemplation in silence on him." (see source 2 p. 102 vers 6.23)

The second quotation is from the Amrita Bindu Upanishad. The word "Self" is used as a synonym for the soul.

"The Om as Word is (fist looked upon as) the Supreme Brahman. After that (word-idea) had vanished, that imperishable Brahman (remains). The wise one should meditate on that imperishable Brahman, if he desires the peace of his soul." (see source 14 verse 16)

The Upanishads date originally from 800-400 BC. There are 112 original Upanishads written in Sanskrit, of which 14 are regarded as being particularly significant (see source 2 p. 7 and source 12 p. 87). Of these the oldest are the most interesting, because they are simple and straightforward. Many writers of later date have also wanted to call their works Upanishads, because their messages have a different status if they are included in the group of Vedic scriptures in this way. But the 112 Upanishads constitute the true ending of the *Vedic literature* itself or *The Scriptures,* as the four Vedas and this supplementary Vedic literature are also called.

To conclude this review of these old scriptures the following little quotation from the Amrita Bindu Upinashad, verse 19, can be useful in placing the texts in their proper perspective [the word "Jnana" is Sanskrit and means knowledge achieved through meditative contact with the divine]:

"Of cows which are of diverse colours
the milk is of the same colour.
(the intelligent one) regards Jnana as the milk,
and the many-branched Vedas as the cows."
(see source 14 verse 19)

The Vedanta Philosophy: everything is oneness

The word "vedanta" itself means "the end of the Vedas". The essence of the Vedanta philosophy is that everything is oneness and that this oneness is the only reality. Human beings are also just a part of the same divine oneness. Therefore, we are living in an illusion if we perceive ourselves as individuals and believe that time and place exist. To acknowledge and experience oneness with everything outside time and space is an important step towards realisation (see source 6 p. 383). The following examples show how simply and beautifully this approach is expressed in the Katha Upanishad, part 2, and in the Maitri Upinashad:

"When the wise realize the omnipresent Spirit, who rests invisible in the visible and permanent in the impermanent, then they go beyon sorrow."
(see source 2 p. 59)

"He who is in the sun, and in the fire and in the heart of man is ONE. He who know this is one with the ONE." (see source 2 p. 101 at the end of vers 6.17)

The Yoga Philosophy: 8 steps to realisation

Patañjali systematised the knowledge from the Vedic literature and created the Yoga system as an entity. He formulated the thoughts in his scriptures, Yoga Sutras, upon which many people and schools of thought have since been based. This is why he is known today as the "father" of the yoga system. Patañjali lived either a couple of hundred years BC or a corresponding period AD. The historians are not agreed, so his lifetime cannot be dated more precisely.

The word "yoga" derives from Sanskrit and means "unification". It lies thus in the word itself that yoga is a method for uniting with the divine (see source 28 p. 9). In its entirety the Yoga system consists of eight steps. The first five deal with moral maxims and physical exercises for maintaining and controlling the body and its functions. The best known in the West is Hatha Yoga which is precisely a combination of elements from these five steps. The sixth step is about concentration. Raja Yoga focuses on the seventh step which deals with, how one can regulate the mind through meditation, while the eighth and final step represents the veritable uniting with God. The word "yoga" is Sanskrit and means "to unite" and in the spiritual context "to unite with the highest being – God". The underlying philosophy in the Yoga system is that a person is not perfect until all eight aspects are mastered

Kali Yuga: our era

If most people today live in the illusion of being separate from the divine, it has something to do with our spiritual era. Indian spiritual philosophy distinguishes between four different spiritual eras: satyayuga, tretāyuga, dvāparayuga and kaliyuga. In the same way as the seasons, they occur in a repeated cycle and each has its own special quality. It takes 4.32 million years to go through such a cycle. At the moment we are in the Kali Yuga which began approximately 5,000 years ago and will continue for another 427,000 years (see source 11 p. 290). The words "kali yuga" mean "dark ages", which in this connection is understood as "the age of ignorance". What we are ignorant of is our divine origin. Indian gurus and wise men knew that most people in this era would live without an acknowledgement and experience of their own divine essence. Therefore they have undertaken to work to bring light into the darkness of this age. The Vedic literature has been and still is one of the instruments for achieving this (see source 6 p. 389).

HINDUISM

The influence of Hinduism throughout the ages

Although Hinduism is the most widespread religion in India (approx. 80 % of the population are Hindus), it is misleading to call it the Indian religion. The second largest religious group is the Muslims (approx. 10 % of the population), and after that come the Christians (approx. 2.7 % of the population), the Buddhists (approx. 0.7 % of the population) etc. – practically every religion is represented in this multifarious country (cf. source 22 p. 73, 77, 78 and 82). Both Hinduism and Buddhism originated here. However, it is quite definitely the Hindu symbols that catch your eye first in the Indian temple chaos. Hinduism has its roots in Vedic religion (see source 7) and is an open religion in the sense that it does not reject other religious persuasions – in fact it arose itself as a collection of many religious traditions in India.

Hinduism is also interesting because it has left deep imprints on the whole culture of the country; partly in the form of the caste system and partly in the belief in reincarnation and that there is a final goal to strive for where the soul becomes free. According to Hinduism, when this goal has been attained, it is no longer necessary to live any more lives as a human being on earth. This kind of salvation can only be attained through a life in cooperation with the gods.

The Hindu teachings are communicated in a both unique and also very elegant manner by the many god figures of the religion who each in their own way reflect various aspects of the divine. Many heroic myths tell of the lives and doings of the gods – stories which can be understood factually and also interpreted on a symbolic level. By means of their roles and deeds they become symbols of human tendencies and possibilities. You bring the aspects you want to develop into your life by reaching out to the god or gods which reflect these. Some gods are more popular than others. It is especially the most popular gods which are depicted and worshipped in the many temples of India and other public places where altars are erected – also in private homes.

There are several reasons why it is interesting to take a closer look at Hinduism. Because it is also in this religion that the concept "bhakti", "devotional love", is defined and identified as the path to the divine goal. The concept of bhakti is introduced in the original Hindu "Bible": the Bhagavadgita. The Bhagavadgita specifies that through the love of one's God – here as a personified God – human beings achieve decisive progress in their striving towards the divine state. In the Bhagavadgita the concrete god was Krishna, but that does not prevent the Hindus from replacing this god with other gods and teachers whom they worship in the same way. In this way the foundation for the people's love for Hinduism's many gods and also for the gurus was laid.

The Bhagavadgita – the Hindu "Bible"

The Indian people, just like other peoples, have old heroic narratives about the ethical and temporal conditions of life. One of the best known works from the oldest Indian literature is the Bhagavadgita poem, which is also just called the Gita. This poem and the Upanishads can more or less be designated as a kind of Bible for the Hindus. However it is known that the Gita originates from around 300 BC, but this scripture is also difficult to date precisely. But it is known that it is younger than the Vedas and some of the Upanishads, because reference is made to these scriptures in the Bhagavadgita. The word "Bhagavad" means the "the Elevated One", and "Gita" means "Song". This can be translated a little freely as "The Word of the Lord". The Lord appears in the poem in the form of the god Krishna who speaks "his words" to the king and the young man Arjuna.

The Bhagavadgita is only a part of the very comprehensive heroic poem, the *Mahabharata,* the plot of which describes the final battle between two branches of the same family. Just as the parties are drawn up before each other and are ready to fight, Arjuna's courage fails him. He is standing on the one side with Krishna and his family, while others of his relations and friends are on the opposing side. Arjuna does not want to kill them and he cannot see that anything at all positive can come out of this unhappy and deadlocked situation. He is therefore in doubt as to whether he should fight at all. It is at this point that Krishna delivers his exhortations, and it is the conversation between Krishna and Arjuna in this scene which constitutes the Bhagavadgita. The poem consists of 18 songs which again are divided up into a number of verses (cf. source 8). Therefore, the references in this and the following chapter are given in the following form: (song number. verse number). There are a number of repetitions in the poems, so the references are only examples of places in the text where the ideas mentioned are expressed.

Precisely at the critical point where everything appears hopeless to Arjuna, Krishna initiates him into the mystery of life. Krishna explains that death is an illusion, because the human soul is immortal. Instead the soul continues in a different dimension when the body dies (2.17-31). He explains that the goal of all humans is to achieve perfection and become one with God. He initiates Arjuna into Yoga which is about letting go of desires and lust, because liberation from these is one of the instruments for achieving realisation (2.39-72 and 3.3-43). These messages are all in accordance with the ideas in the Vedic literature.

The Concept of Bhakti: devotional love

However, what is special in the Bhagavadgita is that Krishna introduces a new method which he presents as *the shortcut* to the highest goal. Unlike the methods which existed at that time, it does not involve renouncing the world. Instead Arjuna is encouraged to live and act in love and devotion to God through all his activities. This is done by carrying out all actions in life as a divine duty offered in devotion to Him. The method is called "bhakti"; the word means "devotion". By linking all costs and gains from our deeds to the God in this way, we free ourselves from personal costs and gains. Thus we also free ourselves from our own desires and needs. Instead our actions will be carried out in accordance with our divine source (5.7-10 and 6.1-4). If everything is done in devotion to God, you do not bear any blame (2.38). Then all actions will lead you to Him (9.26-28). Arjuna is warned that as a warrior he must do his duty and, if necessary, kill others (2.31-33). For we all have an innate duty to be fulfilled which we should not opt out of, (18.47-48 and 4.34). Bound by this duty, we also have to do things we may not wish to do in order not to perish (18.60). But if everything is done with God in mind, we can achieve the highest goal even though the act involves killing relatives (12.6-8). By doing our duty we are just an instrument doing what the Lord has already decided (11.33 and 18.60-61). In the course of the conversation Krishna reveals his true nature to Arjuna. In this way Arjuna learns that Krishna truly is God (11.5-55) and that this god is eternally present in everything (18.12-15 and 9.29-32).

Thus by introducing the concept of Bhakti which defines love for the personified god as the true path to attaining the divine goal, Krishna breaks with the sacrificial tradition of the Vedas. He states quite unequivocally that realisation cannot be achieved via theoretic studies of the scriptures. Realisation and attainment of the divine goal are described in the Gita as seeing the true form of Krishna and coming to him. To Arjuna he says (11.52-55):

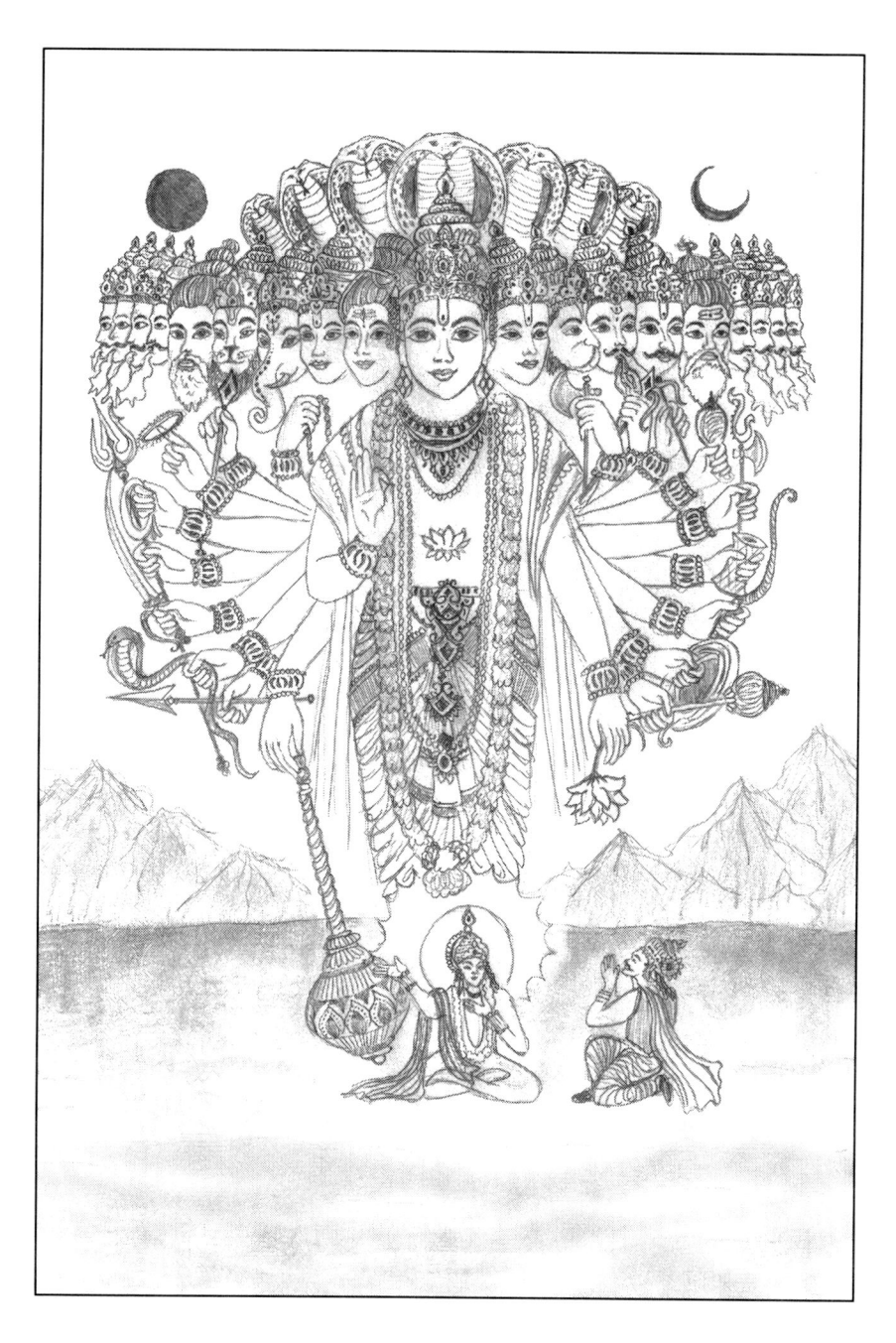

Lord Krishna granted Arjuna divine eyes by which he could see Krishna in his Universal Form. Drawing: Signe Emine Petersen

"This form of Mine (with four arms) which you have just seen is exceedingly difficult to perceive. Even the gods are always eager to behold this form.

Neither by study of the Vedas nor by penance, nor again by charity, nor even by ritual can I be seen in this form (with four arms) as you have seen Me.

Through single-minded devotion, however, I can be seen in this form (with four arms), nay, known in essence and even entered into, O valiant Arjuna.

Arjuna, he who performs all his duties for My sake, depends on Me, is devoted to Me: has no attachment, and free from malice towards all beings, reaches Me."

Just as the parables in the Bible can be interpreted at several levels, the storyline in the Bhagavadgita can be regarded as an illustration of the struggle within ourselves. Before the battle, Arjuna chose Krishna as his charioteer. Figuratively speaking, this shows that he chose the divine power to steer his energy and behaviour. Parts of Krishna's message can be interpreted in the following way: We should do our duty and follow the divine will, trusting that this power – the charioteer in the poem – will lead us on the right path. In source 33 page 248 the view is put forward that what happened between Krishna and Arjuna was not actually a conversation. Because at this decisive moment in the combat, when the parties were about to fight the battle, there was no time at all to say all the words contained in the Gita. Instead Krishna raised the young man to a higher state of spiritual consciousness in which the truth was revealed in a few moments for Arjuna within himself so that he himself attained the realisation of the Gita's wisdom.

For us in the West it is worth noticing that the aim of this devotional love is not towards a gain for the god or the guru, but for the person submitting him or herself in love to the god or the guru. In this case it is Arjuna who will harvest the gain if he carries out all his actions in remembrance of Krishna. It will bring Arjuna into contact with the higher vibration for which Krishna is an expression.

In India there has always been a tradition for spiritual teachers, and the Gita's call to live in love for a personified god, Krishna, has also opened up for support for the work of the others. Even though the Hindus have taken the bhakti-concept of devotion to heart, they do not choose only to worship Krishna. In spite of the fact that Krishna says directly to Arjuna that he is God and that worshipping him is the easiest way to attaining realisation, many Indians have maintained their attachment to many gods from the old scriptures.

Since the time of the Vedas a good many gurus have made a deep impression on the people and made their mark on the traditions and history of the country. Even today it is a natural part of Indian everyday life to offer sacrifices to several of their favourite gods and gurus. The object of their sacrifices depends on what they wish to achieve. In the practice of this religion, rituals and mantras and other Vedic instructions still play an important part. So together the Bhagavadgita and the Vedic literature form the foundation for the Hindu religion and the work of the spiritual gurus. For Hindus believe that by sacrificing to certain gods, they focus on the energies within themselves which these gods represent. Thus the god symbols in the external world are of great importance for one's own work on the inner level. In this way both the gods and the concepts are interwoven in the broad embrace of Hinduism.

The symbolic language of Hinduism

When I arrived in India, I knew very little about the Vedas and even less about Hinduism. On my previous trip I just had to admit that the brilliantly coloured Hindu temples with their over decorated statues did not attract me at all. I did not immediately understand why their gods often had several heads and many arms and why parts of their bodies were replaced by animal limbs. The whole menagerie seemed to me to be a little naive and silly. In reality I was the naive one, because

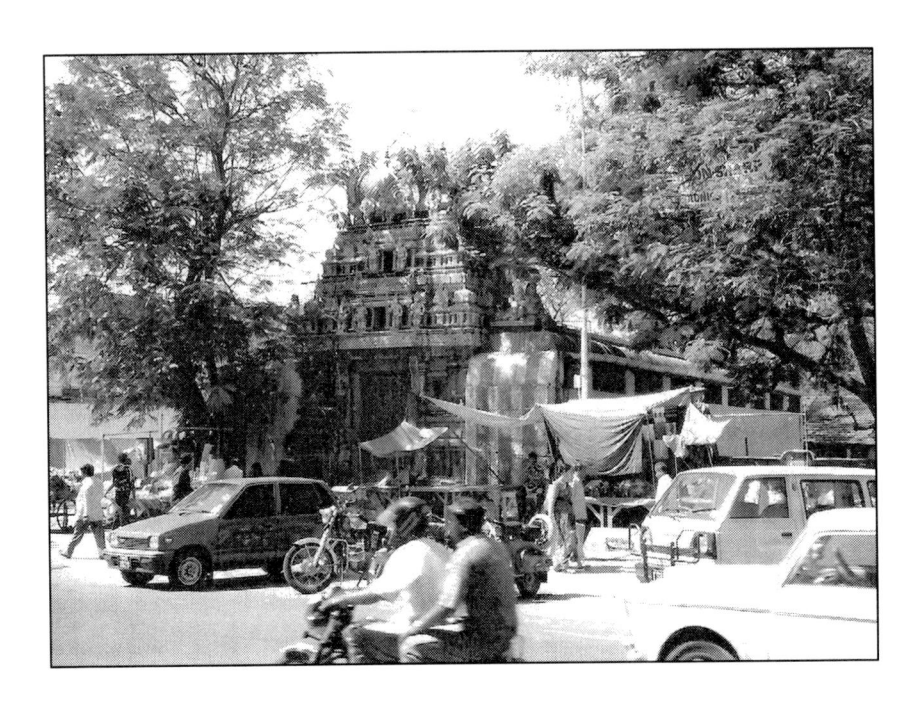

As this example shows, some temples are also situated in the centre of the town. Photo: Lennart Nordstrand

I realised later that every little detail on these figures has a symbolic meaning, originating from a deep insight into human nature. I met a German philosopher while visiting one of the gurus. He aroused my interest in how parts of the Indian spiritual philosophy are expressed through the symbolism of the nature and actions of the Hindu gods.

As mentioned, the goal for a Hindu is to become a perfect human being – that is to become one with his or her divine nature. When this is achieved, the door is opened to a life in a new dimension. Until then, humans are subject to the principle of reincarnation in which one is constantly attached to birth, life, death, new rebirth, life, death – and so on – in the wheel of life. But by acknowledging and surmounting the weaknesses of human nature, the individual can realise his or her own divine nature. It is during this process towards attaining the divine goal that the many thousands of gods come into the picture. Each one can be interpreted as a symbol of the various aspects of human nature. The appearance of the gods also contributes to render the inner qualities visible which the individual god represents. Furthermore, the origin and mutual relations of the gods are also significant factors which are a part of defining what they represent. By considering the gods and the stories of them with this in mind, one can only feel humility in the face of the wisdom and insight into human nature which is communicated in this brilliant and elegant manner. The following chapters will show how impressively the enormous information about the inner qualities can be communicated by the sound and image symbolism in the outer appearance of a god figure.

The Image Symbolism of the Elephant God

The name Elephant God refers to the physical form of this figure – a human body with an elephant's head. "A rose by any other name …" Ganapati or Ganesh is the best known name for this god. The reason I am choosing to describe the symbolism for Ganapati is partly because of his popularity and partly because one of the gurus I visited is also called Ganapati (see the chapter on the gurus). Background knowledge about the Elephant God will make it easier to understand the meaning of this guru's name and role.

Ganapati is the son of the god Shiva and his wife Parvati. One version of the story of Ganapati tells that Shiva chopped his original head off in ignorance of the fact that the boy was his son. Shiva had been away for many years and had never seen his son who, therefore, did not know his father either. Ganapati had been given the task of guarding his mother's house. Because of the boy's courage and fighting spirit, Shiva had to finally behead him in order to gain access to Parvati. When he realised whom he had killed, he ordered his men to bring him the head of the

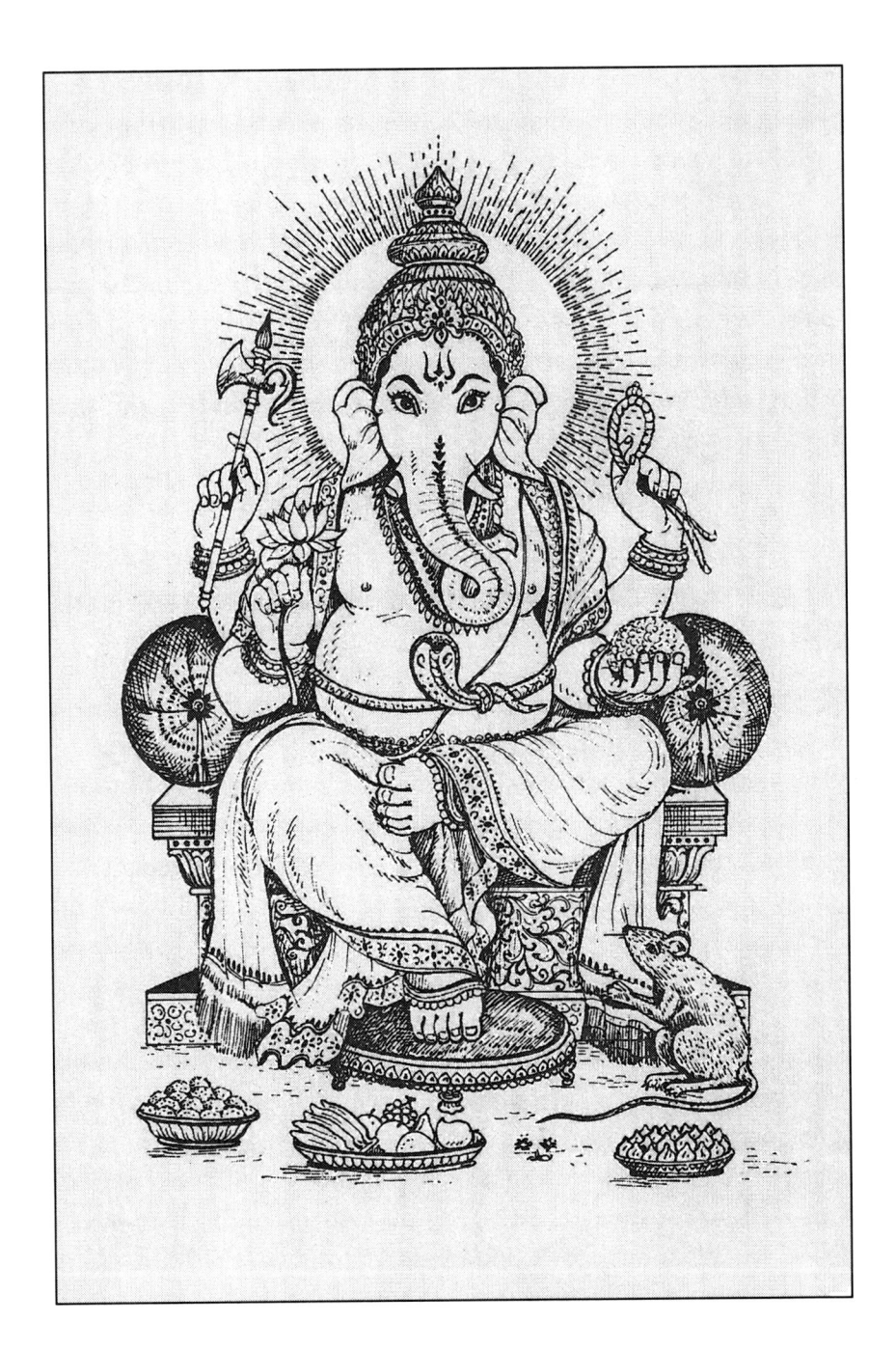

Ganapati/Ganesh. See source information II

first creature they met on their way. It turned out to be an elephant whose head the boy was given as a replacement. He was brought to life again and has since worn this head (see source 15, figure 37).

Today Ganapati is the symbol of intelligence, wisdom and abundance. He is the god who can remove any obstacle, and he is often seen as the guardian of a whole town. People often sacrifice to him because they believe that it will make them better at acquiring wisdom or increase their possibilities for achieving success in business.

Ganapati's nature and his special characteristics are shown symbolically by his form and stance. The following will reveal how superbly and precisely this can be done:

The name itself already tells a lot about this Elephant God, because both "Ganapati" and "Ganesh" mean "Lord of all Beings" in Sanskrit – the old, sacred language. When trying to understand how these abilities and this position can be attributed to Ganapati, it is most obvious to look at his origins. For upon his creation he was given equal parts of his parents' natures. The father, Shiva, who is described in more detail in the following chapter, knows the origin of all things and thus represents "the highest being". The mother, Parvati, is the symbol of the "giver of energy" which is necessary for activating any thought and action. Together they form the whole: all knowledge as well as the ability to activate actions. As Ganapati has inherited this insight and energy, he is destined to be "lord over all beings". For he has experienced and understood his existence and his divine origin, and by virtue of the energy from his mother he can act on the basis of this wisdom.

If a god were to be pictured in the form of an ordinary human being, there is a limit to how many characteristics such a figure can illustrate. But giving Ganapati an elephant's head indicates that he possesses some of the characteristics of the elephant. Among other things, elephants are known for their intelligence and good memory which are precisely the characteristics of Ganapati. The large ears are a symbol of the fact that Ganapati has listened to and heard the divine truth. Combined with intelligence this means that he has also reflected on and understood this truth. This makes him the symbol of divine wisdom. The trunk of the elephant is a quite unique instrument, because it can handle tiny as well as enormous things with the same precision. The fact that this instrument is placed on the head tells that Ganapati's intellect masters both the coarse material world as well as the spiritual world which is finer in substance. The trunk is formed like a circle in order to show that he can make the round AUM sound with which the universe was created. The last peculiarity of Ganapati's elephant head is the tusks, one of which is broken. The paired tusks symbolise the antithesis of all things between which we humans are caught, heat-cold, sorrow-joy, day-night etc. The fact that one tusk is broken shows that Ganapati is no longer retained in this world of antithesis, but lives beyond these trivialities. He rests in the divine truth.

Ganapati's large stomach symbolises the fact that he holds the whole universe within himself. The stomach and the intestines are the organs in which we absorb and digest our food. Ganapati's stomach is so big that it can absorb and digest every experience and idea in the universe. The snake around his stomach is an image of the kundalini force. It is the basic energy which we normally neither know nor use, but which rests at the base of our spine. The fact that Ganapati has tied the snake around his stomach shows that he not only knows but also masters this force.

The stance of the legs and feet is also significant. Ganapati is sitting on a chair. One leg is bent naturally and the foot is resting on the floor. The other leg is bent outwards so this foot is resting on the opposite thigh as with a meditating yogi. This shows that he has a foothold in this physical world on the earth as well as having his awareness in the divine in meditation. Around the feet of the god there is an abundance of food. This shows that he has everything. The rat at his feet is sitting waiting for Ganapati's permission to eat. The rat is the symbol of greed, because the nature of this animal is to keep gathering to itself, even though it cannot eat any more food. The fact that the rat here has subjected itself to Ganapati's will shows that Ganapathi himself has overcome and mastered all desires.

Ganapati has four arms. The objects which he holds in his hands underline further the properties which he masters. In one hand he holds an axe which he has used to break the connection to every desire. With the rope he has pulled himself out of the turmoil of this world in order just to rest in the divine love. He also holds a bowl of rice. This represents the reward which the spiritual seeker achieves at the goal. His last hand is holding a lotus flower which is the symbol of the perfect goal for human development – becoming one with God. The special quality of the lotus flower is that it often grows in dirty lakes and marsh holes. When it unfolds its petals, it reveals the most beautiful flower which is both pure and white and completely unaffected by the impurities of its surroundings. With this symbol the god Ganapati shows us humans both the journey and the goal; when we live our lives focussing on our inner selves, the most beautiful flower – the divine goal – will unfold at our journey's end (see source 16, page 8-15).

Considering all this information, Ganapati becomes a symbol of human deification. He shows us which characteristics to use to overcome all challenges within ourselves in order for us, like the lotus flower, to find our way through the temptations of the mind and the conditions of our lives without becoming a part of these inner and outer circumstances. Seen in this light it is completely understandable, that Ganapati is such a popular figure all over India.

The "Infinite Universe" – Brahma, Vishnu and Shiva

The most difficult part of any religion is creating a connection to the abstract and infinite, the unlimited and intangible god concept: "The Infinite Universe". As a rule the connection between the "known and comprehensible" and the "infinite and indescribable" is made via more tangible figures which we as humans can relate to more easily. In Hinduism the three gods, Brahma, Vishnu and Shiva constitute this connection. This makes them the most important gods, because they are the ones closest to the infinite source. Since the "Infinite Universe" in this context is an expression which designates what has no beginning or end, because it has always existed and will continue to do so – it is that which includes absolutely *everything*. In order to try to grasp this Infinite Universe, the Hindus divide it into these three groups of principles which exist in all the aspects of the universe: the creative, the preserving and the destructive principle. All things – except infinity – contain a beginning, a preservation and a dissolution. The three gods are each assigned their own principle. Thus Brahma represents the creative aspect, Vishnu the preserving and Shiva the destructive aspect – i.e. letting go of the old to make way for a new beginning. In Hinduism the Infinite Universe is called "Brahman" (see source 24, p. 11). Note that the god Brahma and the Infinite Universe, Brahman, ending in "n" instead of "a", are two different things, although the words are similar.

Although Brahma represents the creative principle, he himself was born from a lotus flower which grew out of the navel of Vishnu. Therefore the two argue about who actually came first. But nobody created Shiva, for he has always been. The mystery of his creation commands the respect of the two other gods which gives Shiva the highest status of the three.

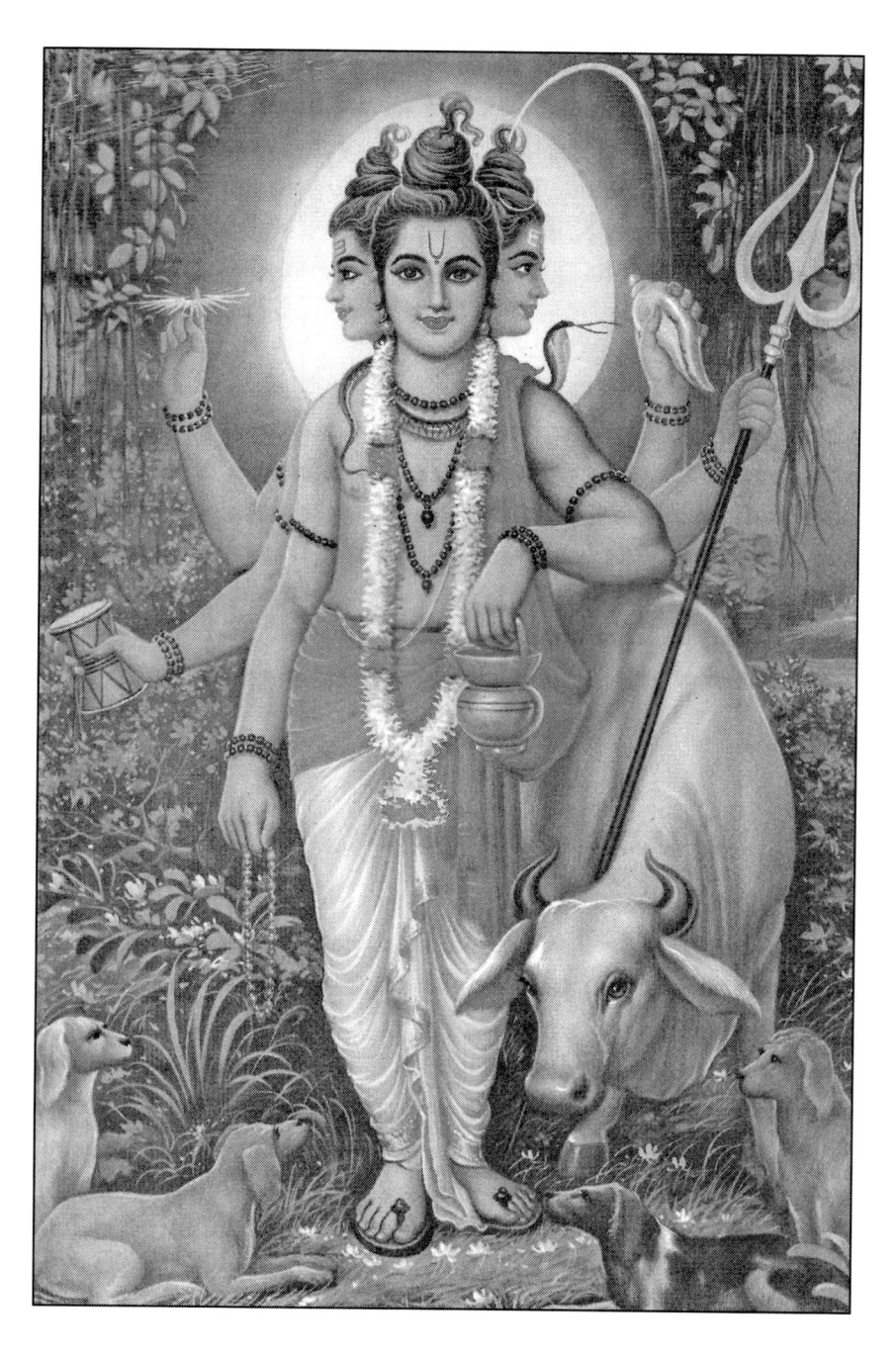

Dattatreya: Brahma, Vishnu and Shiva. See source information III

According to Hinduism Brahma, Vishnu and Shiva have each let themselves be reincarnated on earth several times. This principle of reincarnation is one of the key elements in Hinduism, which make it possible for this religion to relate with tolerance towards other religions. For example, the god Krishna is said to be the eighth incarnation of Vishnu, while Buddha is believed to be his ninth incarnation (see source 6, p. 364-366). In this way the whole Buddhist religion becomes a small branch of Hinduism.

On a special occasion the three gods were incarnated in one and the same person: Dattatreya. He is pictured as a human being with one body and three heads. This illustrates that the three god aspects are just different aspects of the same whole. As Dattatreya in this way constitutes *the whole*, he is the symbol of the guru who can tell humans about the highest: Brahman. It is said of the guru Swamiji, one of the four I visited, that he is an incarnation of Dattatreya.

Yantra – Geometric Symbols

In India, many paths have been tried to reach out for and unfold the spiritual truths of the universe. There are numerous methods and instructions as to how human beings can achieve this divine state. The use of mantras and ritual ceremonies with god figures which represent humans with some animal limbs are examples of this. But in order to round off this Indian world of symbols, we must not forget the third type of symbols: yantra. A yantra is a geometric figure created by using endless circles and lines. It can be both 2 and 3 dimensional. In their own quite peculiar symbolic way these yantras can illustrate the spiritual truths and contexts.

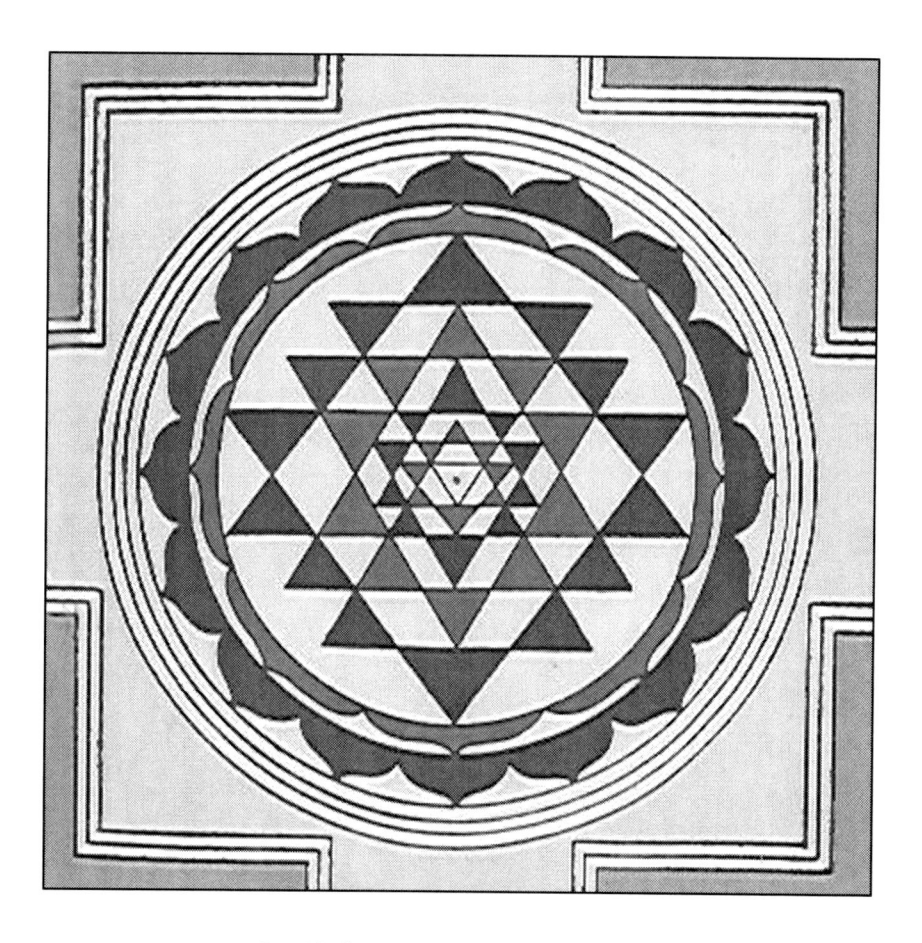

Sri Chakra. See source information IV

One of the best known yantras is called "Sri Chakra". With its triangles, circles, lines and not least the dot in the middle – called bindu – shows the whole Universe and its contexts (see source 24, p. 15). Among others, it is the figure with which the guru Swamiji performed rituals every morning. See Figure 7A which shows the yantra Sri Chakra.

INDIA TODAY – THE LAND OF CONTRASTS

There is something for all the senses

Considering the religious background of this country, it might be expected that humanity and compassion would play a marked role in the everyday life of the Indian people. This is apparently not the case! It is probably a remnant from the heyday of the caste system that many rich Indians treat the poor like animals, while they pander to each other. The rich are very rich, and the poor live at or even below subsistence level. In fact it is said that no Indians would starve if the wealth of the rich Indians were to be distributed among all the people in this country.

On the streets contrasts are to be seen everywhere: The dreary greyish-brown streets with the dust and the ramshackle huts are in strong contrast to the bright and beautiful colours shining towards you from the clean and well-dressed Indian women. The doorman at the posh hotels with his clean, white gloves is in deep contrast to the reek of the city. The fat Indians are extremely fat, the slim are correspondingly emaciated. With some you meet unbounded helpfulness, with others an impertinence which is both tiring and unpleasant. With many of those who have daily dealings with tourists, the attitude is: if you can get away with it, it's ok. In contrast to this I also experienced being invited to a wedding by a fellow passenger on a plane who was a stranger to me. An event which lasted two days, all expenses paid.

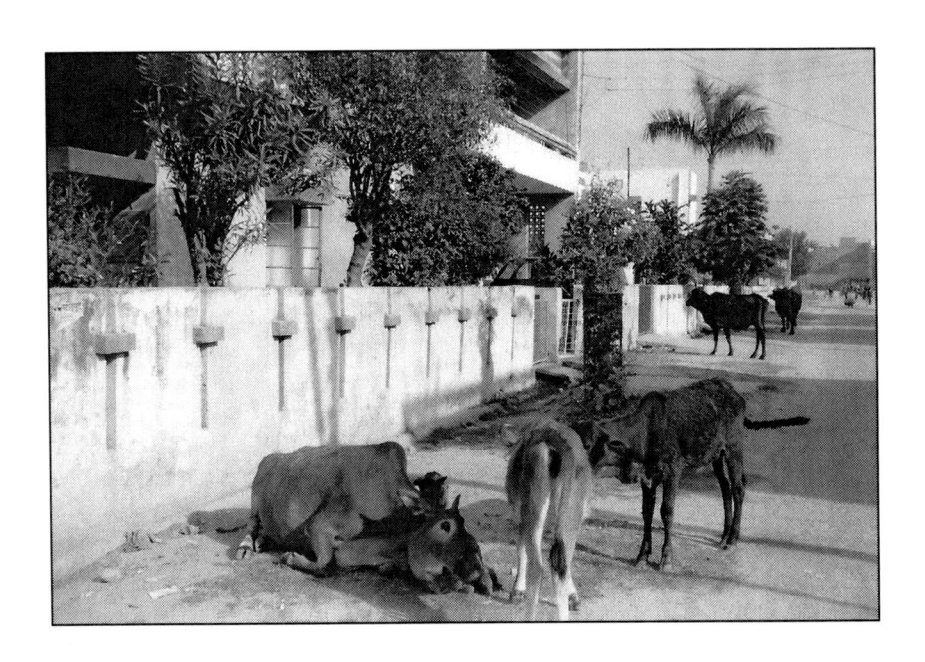

Cows in the street in Lucknow. Photo: Lisbeth Ejlertsen

And I could go on like this ... One thing which always makes me wonder is how relatively drab the Indian middle class homes are – seen with Danish eyes. In our culture, decorating our homes is a priority which is often higher than decorating ourselves. I wonder how it is that Indian people, whose way of dressing beautifully and wearing jewellery is mastered to perfection, can be so indifferent about their home environment. Perhaps this complete lack of logic is one of the things which make a visit to India fascinating.

Being in India is a total experience. You cannot stay there without having all your senses bombarded: You are confronted with smells ranging through everything from faeces to perfumed incense. At times it can be difficult to decide which is worst. Everywhere the contrasts between poverty and wealth are visible. Your hearing is overwhelmed by the intense noise level of the cities contrasting deeply with the quietness of many of the temples. The food assaults your taste buds with everything from the hottest chilli to the sweetest confectionary. Finally, the burning sun with its massive heat feels like a complete contrast to the air-conditioned rooms which by comparison feel very much like refrigerators.

Maybe it is because it is so overwhelming to be in this country that one is forced to find the quiet place within oneself and just rest there in order to stand it. This seems to be what the Indians do. That is why they seem so calm and relaxed as a rule, even though everything around them is chaos. It is very fascinating! To live like this in inner peace and rest there regardless of the unrest in the outer world, that was and is one of my goals.

A SPECIAL PALM LEAF ASTROLOGER

A little about astrologers and palm leaf astrologers

The basis for the science of astrology is the idea that the stars and planets in our solar system affect the lives of human beings. Throughout time special qualities have been assigned to the sun, moon, planets and star constellations. The astrologers map out the relative positions of the stars and planets in the sky and construct a horoscope which they then can decipher and interpret. It is particularly interesting to study the position of the celestial bodies at the time of a person's birth, because this reveals the qualities which the person received at birth as gifts. In the course of a person's life, the planets move across the Zodiac in the sky. The Zodiac consists of 12 animal star constellations which we call Star Signs. As time passes and the celestial bodies move, the degree of influence of each of them changes. It is possible to calculate the positions of the planets at a given point in time. Using the birth horoscope as a reference, it is possible to determine at any time the energies which will affect that person. Thus the science of astrology can give guidelines for a whole lifetime, and the astrologer can make pronouncements about both the past and the future. India was among the first countries to make use of the science of astrology. The Rishis, the spiritually gifted people of India, made use of astrology several thousand years BC.

Palm leaf astrologers do not necessarily have the same qualifications as the "ordinary" astrologers. Instead they communicate the work of their forefathers. The palm leaf astrologers have access to archives of palm leaves on which the fate of various people was written down approximately 3,000 years ago. The palm leaves in question have been conserved and treated so that the information could be scratched on the surface. The text on the palm leaves was dictated at that time by the Rishis who also predicted the fates of some people in our time – several thousand years after their own life on earth.

Before this trip to India I did not know much about palm leaf astrologers. I had once read about the phenomenon in a newspaper article. In this it said that a palm leaf astrologer knew when a person would arrive at their place. The reason is that these leaves which were made several thousand years ago carry both the names of these present-day people and also the time at which they will come and receive the information. These incredible statements had aroused my interest and scepticism. Could it be true that these palm leaves had survived for so many years? Before I left on my trip, I found out that there was a palm leaf astrologer both in New Delhi and in Bangalore, and that the palm leaf archives in both places consist of copies on paper and are thus not real palm leaves. The papers at both places are filed according to the time and place of the person's birth. Therefore, this information has to be given at the start in order to enable the astrologers to find the right paper with the printed predictions. But according to the article, there were also other types of palm leaf astrologers and palm leaf archives in India. I was interested in doing more research on this phenomenon. Equipped only with this small background knowledge, I took my first step out on to the Indian astrology market.

My first experience with an Indian Palmist

After having travelled around with the Guru Swamiji, (cf. the chapter on gurus), I found myself in Chennai (previously called Madras) with a few days to spare. I was impatient and hooked on the idea of palm leaf astrologers, and as neither New Delhi nor Bangalore were among my first destinations, I fancied investigating the possibilities on my own. With the help of a local guide I found out that there was an *Astrologer and Palmist* in town. To think that there was one in Chennai too ...! I immediately decided to phone and arrange a visit.

Soon afterwards I was sitting in his dark office with the red lighting and looking at the many gold rings on his fingers. He wanted to look at the palms of my hands and began his predictions while I sat impatiently waiting for him to fetch the real palm leaves. Then he suddenly asked me to turn off the tape recorder I had brought with me, after which he made unpleasant remarks about the curses of previous lives which would cause illness and other devilry in this life. And it would cost around a thousand dollars if he were to neutralise these curses with prayers and magic. I was quite dumbfounded at the turn the séance had taken, and we agreed to take a break while the astrologer saw the next client. It was a fellow traveller that I had met at one of the gurus'. We were not allowed to be present at each other's séances, but even so it felt good that he was sitting there in the next room. He ended up by rescuing me when much later I was sitting with the astrologer again and was once more feeling confused about what was going on. For my fellow traveller put his head round the door with just the right timing and told me in Danish to get out and take my money with me. Soon after we got away from there without paying more than the normal basic rate. It wasn't until then that I realised that the word "palm" in this context means the flat of your hand and has nothing whatsoever to do with palm leaves. A palmist reads palms and, therefore, the man was just doing his job when he was looking at my hands and making his predictions. The results he arrived out did not have much relation to reality – so that's what can happen if one is too eager for exciting experiences. I came away the richer in experience and luckily only a little poorer.

The Meeting with the Special Palm Leaf Astrologer

It was a palm leaf astrologer, who was completely unknown to me before this journey, who made the greatest impression and seemed the most convincing. In a small centre in Vaitheeswaran Koil on the south coast of India I had the experience of my life. The palm leaves here were real palm leaves and they were special, because they were filed according to thumb prints. This means that the absolutely only information required to find the right palm leaf from the archives was a thumb print. This astrologer's leaves are completely personal, as not only are they connected to a thumb print, but they also contain the *name* of the owner. I was curious to visit the astrologer to see the whole scenario, but most of all I was excited to know, whether there might be a palm leaf with my name on it.

Feeling a little unwell with the remains of a fever in my body, I stood outside the astrologer's door on this morning. The town was small, dingy and poor. Although it was only nine o'clock in the morning, there were already 10-12 people waiting there. It was a Sunday and I had been in doubt as to whether he would be open. But I was lucky as Wednesday was the weekly day off in this place. As a lone Western woman with all my kit, I naturally attracted attention. After having had my thumb print taken, I was guided down into the furthest and coolest part of the room, where two other Indian men were waiting for their palm leaves. It turned out that there was not just one astrologer, but four of them each sitting with a client translating information from the palm leaves. So it seemed to me that it was pure translation work on their part, and that they did not make use of special clairvoyant abilities. In this place it was the palm leaf archive itself that was special. The two men who were waiting with me were the only ones who spoke understandable English, so in the course of the next ten hours we became firm friends. It was nice to have their company, because it took all of six hours before it was my turn to take my place at one of the desks.

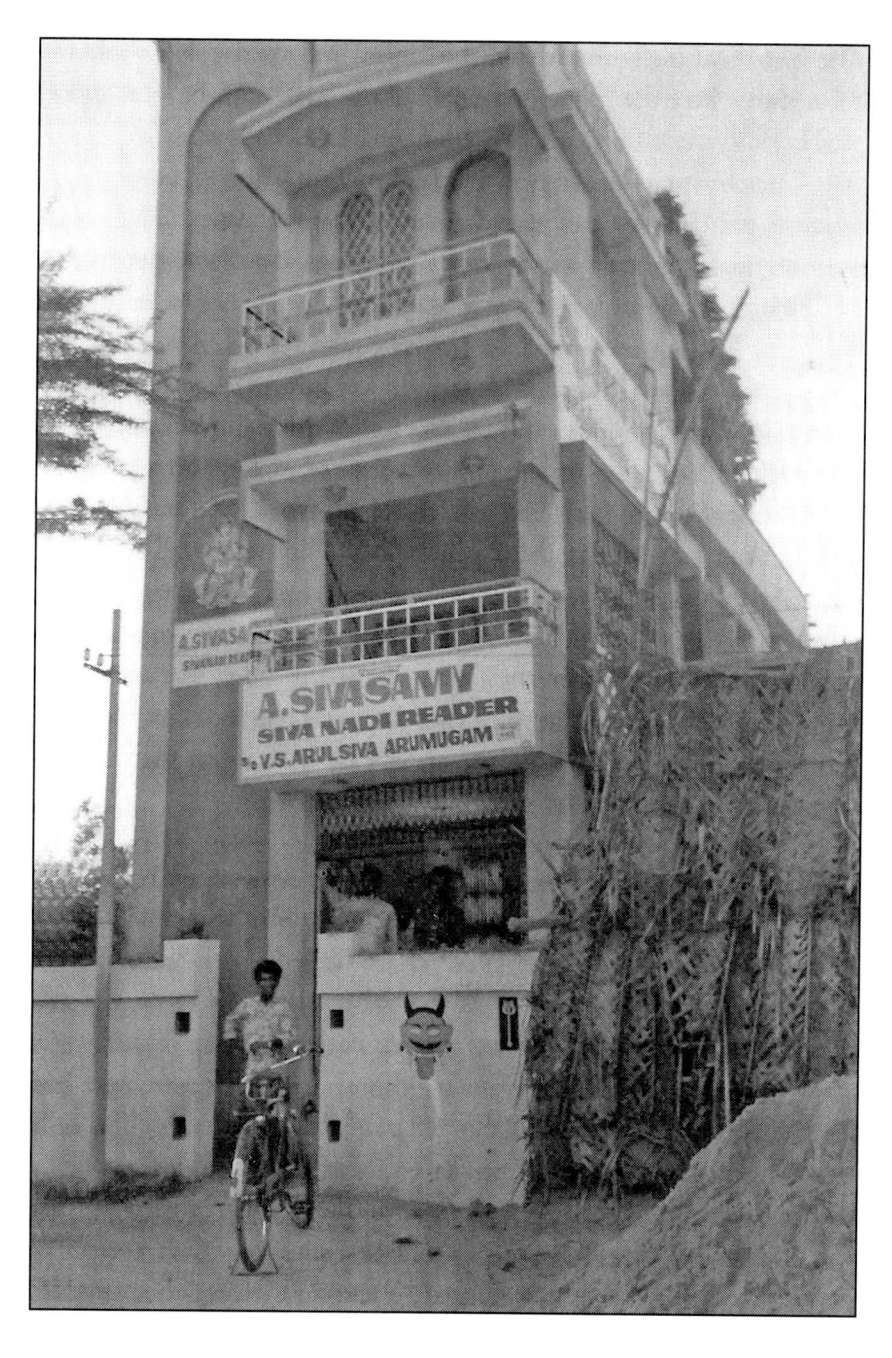

*The office of the palm leaf astrologer A. Sivasamy – note
the house next door ... See source information V*

The historical background for this palm leaf archive is as follows: Palm leaves were the "paper material" of the past, and the astrological predictions were only a part of the information which was filed in this way. Later in time the kings of the Indian Tamil district collected all types of palm leaves and stored them in large libraries. Their texts were originally written in the sacred language, Sanskrit. But a king of Tanjore, who was particularly interested in art and science, had the palm leaves translated into his language, Tamil. Under British sovereignty, the palm leaves with astrological information were bought at auction. The new owner was an ancestor of this palm leaf astrologer. The archive had been in the family's possession for 300 years, and the palm leaf centre itself had existed for 80 years. The business was at this time run by the third generation. The owner calls himself Nadi Astrologer. The word "nadi" means "at the right time". This refers to the fact that the clients will come and get the information on their palm leaves when they have reached precisely the age which is specifically stated on the palm leaf. So it was predicted on the palm leaves themselves how old the person will be when he or she turns up to receive the palm leaf information.

As I had been allowed to be present at the séances with my new Indian friends, I was prepared for what was about to happen, when it was my turn to sit in the "hot" chair. Together we had to check whether my name was on one of the palm leaves. To be on the safe side, I deliberately told the two friends nothing about myself while we were waiting. Based solely on my thumb print, the astrologer had fetched four bundles with about 50 palm leaves in each. The only possible method of selection was to go through all 200 leaves one by one and check whether the information on the leaves matched my life. I only had to answer the astrologer's questions with correct or incorrect, because I was not allowed to reveal anything about myself. For example, they could read from one leaf that my mother had four sisters. As this was incorrect, the leaf was put aside and a new piece of information was read out from the next leaf. This process took a couple of hours besides a lunch break of another hour.

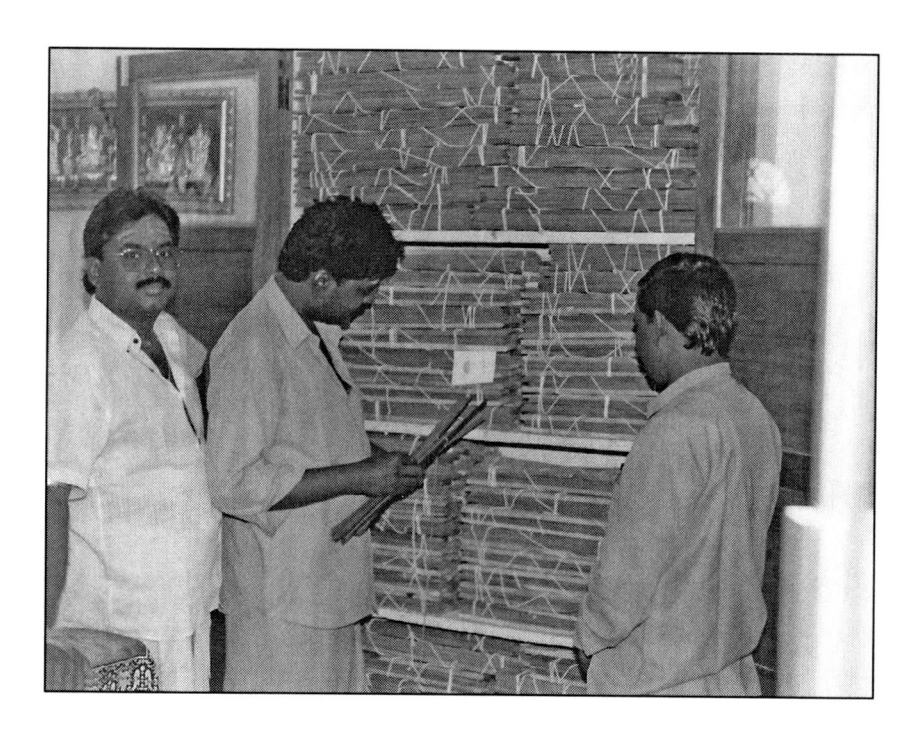

The palm leaf astrologer A. Sivasamy and two employees in front of a filing cabinet with bundles of palm leaves. See source information V

It is time consuming, strenuous and exhausting, when the astrologer has to translate the information from a palm leaf to his local language and another has to translate into English. Then I have to think in Danish, phrase my answers in English after which they have to return by the same route. I was afraid that language misunderstandings might cause my leaf to be laid aside by mistake. When there were only about five of the 200 leaves left, I had given up on the idea that my leaf would be among the rest. But suddenly I became attentive. Two pieces of information on the same leaf were correct. In his hopeless English, the astrologer then stammered out my Danish first and last name from his seat behind the large desk. I was dumbfounded! He continued to state the names of my parents which were also written on the leaf. In order to convince all parties that what he was reading out actually was written on the leaf, the astrologer called one of his colleagues who also read my name out loud. This man could not have followed our conversation, because he had been sitting behind a glass wall in this noisy room and had been busy with his client. There was absolutely no doubt that this palm leaf was *mine*. The other visitors began to gather round our table. Great was their astonishment that the astrologer had had their leaf, but that there also was one for a foreigner like me was beyond their comprehension and mine!

The Appearance of the Palm Leaves

The palm leaves are about four cm in width and about 30 cm in length. They are nougat-brown in colour and quite stiff like thin pieces of wood, almost like veneer. But their surface felt soft, almost as if they had been waxed. A bundle of about 50 palm leaves is protected on top and underneath by a piece of wood. The two pieces of wood and the palm leaves each have two holes through which a long piece of string is threaded. When the string is loosened, the bundle falls apart, but is still held in the right order by the loose string. In this way it is easy for astrologer to leaf through from one palm leaf to another without changing the order.

The writing on a palm leaf has been scratched on to the surface with a sharp instrument. The printed words on the upper and under side of the leaves are as tiny as these printed letters. If the astrologer has difficulty in reading one of the words, he puts a little ink on his finger and spreads it on the writing so that it stands out more clearly. All the basic information about the person in question is written on one leaf. If you want more information, for example about previous lives, they have to find one or more extra palm leaves based on this basic leaf. During my visit, there was no time to find more of my leaves, but I asked for some information to be sent on to me.

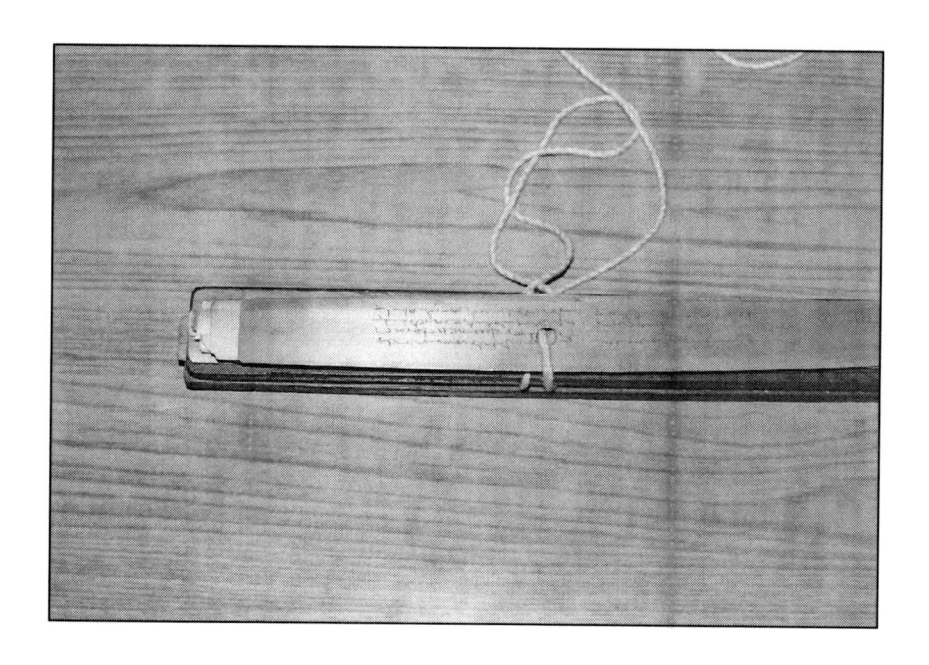

Part of a bundle of long palm leaves with writing. See source information V

About the information on my palm leaf

The story of my meeting with my palm leaf may seem incredible. That is my own feeling, but then again I did actually experience the whole thing. And it was not just a dream. My witnesses are my cassette tape and the little notebook given to me by the astrologer. I had gone alone and unannounced to this place and had spent the night at a hotel 50 km away. Therefore, they could only have had the information about me there which I myself had given them, and that was just my thumb print. During the whole time, I had my passport in a purse around my stomach so nobody could see it. Moreover, it did not hold all the information which the astrologer gave me. My experience with the astrologer in Chennai had taught me to let others talk and keep my own mouth shut. I could only do that until it opened in complete amazement. With the best will in the world my logical sense could find no arguments to disprove what I had experienced. In spite of my great scepticism and wariness, I had to accept what was happening and I could hardly wait to get a translation of the rest of the writing on this interesting leaf.

In addition to my name and those of my parents, it said how many brothers and sisters I had and how many my mother had. The astrologer could tell me how old I was at the time and the day, and the exact date, month and year of my birth. Not only was it predicted more than 3,000 years ago that I would be living on the earth right now, but also that I would be in India and have this information read out to me at this point in my life. It was almost unimaginable. Other information of the leaf was: that I was a foreigner, that I belonged to the Christian faith, that I had an academic, technical education, that I had a special relationship with art, my present job situation, that both my parents were living, that I myself and my siblings were unmarried at that time as well as a characterisation of my qualities. Strangely enough one of these was that I would always thirst after new knowledge via my own experience and that I would return to India again and again. It was precisely this desire that had driven me to India and to the astrologer and which apparently would entice me to new adventures in the future. All this information was absolutely correct.

One piece of information made a particular impression on me. It said that I had two names, an Indian and a Danish one. That was also correct, as 23 days before this day I had asked an Indian guru for an Indian name. The choice of my new name seemed quite random. But *this Indian name* was also written on the leaf! I thought I was the one who had had the idea and the wish to have an Indian name. So how could it have been written on a palm leaf several thousand years before? What if I had not asked the guru for a new name? Then this information would have been wrong. But at the point in time when I was sitting on the chair with the astrologer, the information was correct. And it was even more fantastic when I realised that there were only 15 days to my next birthday. If I had come 15 days later, the information about my present age would not have been true. This

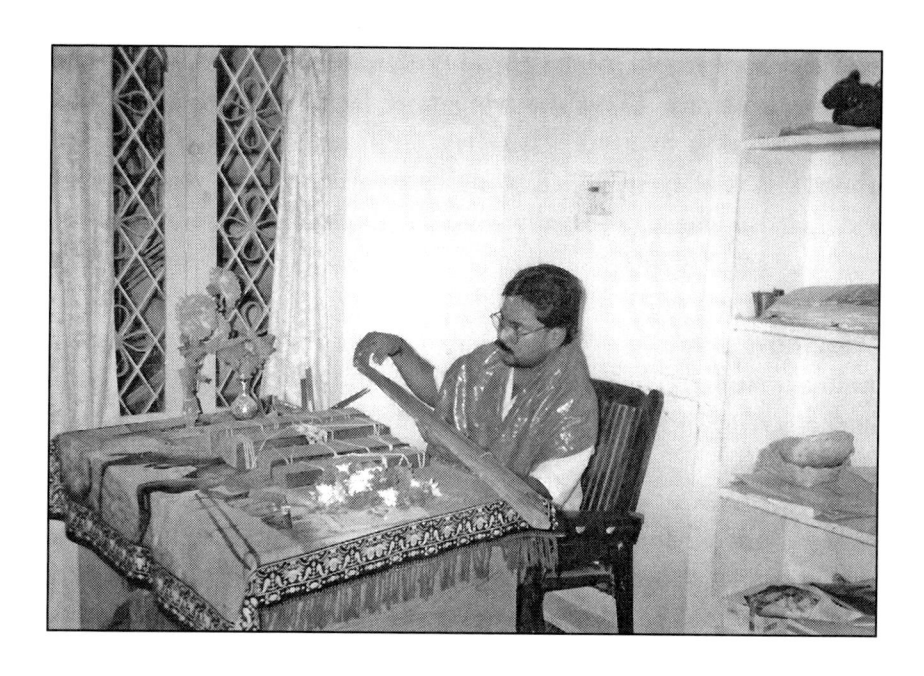

The palm leaf astrologer A. Sivasamy with palm leaf bundles of varying sizes. See source information V

meant that the two pieces of information about my age and my Indian name could only both be correct within an interval of 15 + 23 days. This is not exactly a great margin in view of the fact that the information on the leaf was written approximately 3,000 years before! When I realised this, my remaining defences crumbled. I had to relinquish all resistance and just surrender to this completely crazy and shattering experience. I was both curious and nervous to know what the palm leaf would say about my future.

The information about the future started with a short summary with, among other things, statements about what my financial and health situation would be during the rest of my lifetime. There was information about journeys I would undertake and the kinds of people I would meet on my travels. It also stated which aspects of myself would be fundamental for my future work. After these more general facts followed more specific information of which only a little was given with an exact date in time. For example, the astrologer told me that I would meet a guru in the autumn of 1994 who would give me a mantra. (This did happen; in fact I met two gurus who each gave me a mantra). There was information on the palm leaf about a special event which would take place when I was 49 years old and also what age I finally would reach. At first I found it a little difficult to deal with the last piece of information. However, after reflecting for a while I accepted this information calmly. Seeing as everything else in my life has apparently been planned in such a unique manner, then I am convinced that I will also leave this body at the perfect time.

However, most of the information on the palm leaf was divided up into periods of time, so in this way I was given an insight into the whole course of my life. Among other things, it said that the next 2½ years would be affected by events from previous lives (karma). One of the effects would be that the projects I started would give results, but that the results would be delayed. I immediately became nervous as to whether the next information would be something like what had happened with the previous palmist and be about how much money I would have to pay in order for the karma of previous lives to be eliminated with prayers and rituals. Luckily I was wrong. There was indeed an option to receive information about prayers that would create success, but only if I chose to pay for this information from one of the supplementary palm leaves. As I did not ask for this, the astrologer continued unperturbed to describe the course of life up to the age of 40. Then came information about which factors would be in force from the age of 40-41 and for the periods 41-43 years, 43-50 years, 50-53 years and generally after the age of 50.

One piece of information was about the reactions to what I would write when I got back from India. "Writing" was not at all what I normally engaged in. I had no previous experience as a writer and no ambitions in this direction. But before leaving for India, I had unsuccessfully contacted a few newspapers to hear whether they might be interested in travel accounts from India. I only took this initiative in

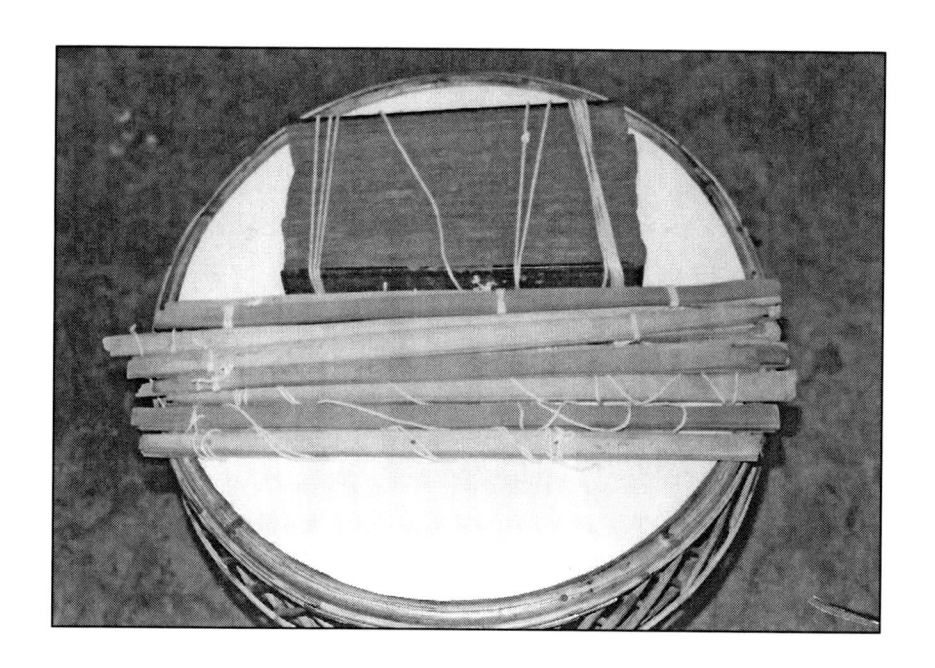

Palm leaf bundles of various sizes on a round table. See source information V

order to perhaps cover some of the costs of the journey. The astrologer could not know anything about this initiative. However, due to all these quite special experiences – particularly at the astrologer's – I ended up with a feeling almost of obligation to pass on this image of "another reality" to others. So when I got home, I did starting writing some material which I tried to have published in 1994. In spite of my persistent attempts, I did not succeed. The result finally came in the form of this book several years later and was thus delayed – as predicted.

In my mind there is no doubt that the following two pieces of information at this palm leaf astrologer's were especially important to me – in fact they were worth the whole visit, regardless of all the other information and predictions:

One of these pieces of information was the clear statement on the palm leaf that "the spiritual element would always be the most important thing in my life". I had never seen myself from without in this light.

But when this characteristic was given so unequivocally, I could feel recognition deep in my heart – and that is actually the way things are in me. It felt as if a couple of cogwheels inside me, which up until that point in time had been moving round each on their own track, had suddenly clicked into place and become synchronised. Suddenly I could understand why I had never felt "at home" in any group, even though I had tried to the best of my ability. As it had never completely succeeded, I had accepted that life would probably be like that for me. With this information a lot of things fell into place inside me – now I knew in which direction to seek in order to find my kind of people. For the best communities are created when people with a common interest come together around the precise subject that they are passionate about. All these inner feelings and reasonings took place in the space of few seconds when the palm leaf astrologer gave me this information.

The other piece of information, which at that time was amazingly important to me, was that I would give birth to a son when I was 37 or 38 years old. Since early childhood I had longed for and looked forward to the day when I should become a mother myself. I had been feeling ready for many years, but fate had decided otherwise. In connection with this I had experienced the great sorrow that due to some health issues it did not seem that this wish would be granted in this life. But with this information my hope was reawakened and also my confidence that this would probably come to pass. Because when all my data and the palm leaf information about my past matched so well, then I dared to open up for the idea that perhaps I might experience the great joy of becoming a mother in spite of everything. My heart was filled with joy and love – and also a little disappointment that it would apparently not be until at least in three years' time if I was to trust the time stated on the palm leaf. But my patience had been in process for many years, so in spite of everything I was prepared to shift my attention so it calmed down at the pleasure of expectation. The leaf also contained an outline of how my future son would fare in his life. It looked bright and promising!

There were also some other interesting predictions on my palm leaf. But as they also concern the future which at the moment of writing I have yet to meet, I will wait to disclose them until time shows whether they come true.

Listen to a little of the recording from the session

[2017: On the book's home page you can hear an excerpt from the session with the palm leaf astrologer which I recorded during my visit. Use the following link or scan the QR code: www.thespiritualwisdomofindia.com/audio-recording-from-the-palm-leaf-astrologer-session/]

How to make use of this

I will not take the information on the future for granted until reality shows whether the predictions are actually fulfilled. All the same, I am not unaffected by this palm leaf information. It is as if in some areas I have been prepared for what *perhaps* will happen. I feel like the earth which has been ploughed and received the seeds which will later give out shoots and grow. The perspectives which the palm leaf information drew for my future seem overwhelming, but also probable, because there is an accordance between these possibilities and my fundamental characteristics, talents and interests. I feel as if my very essence has been revealed – more precisely than I was able to characterise myself. The predictions were not given as a guideline, so that I could create my future in a way to make the predictions come true. If my life does develop in the way described, it will be because the circumstances just develop in that way. All the same, this experience has changed my life in an indefinable way. One of the reasons is that the information on the leaf touched precisely on the areas of my life about which I sometimes worried. For example, how my family situation would develop, whether my job changes were sensible and whether my great interest in spiritual science was a mad idea that I should not focus so much on. I could feel relieved and affirmed on all counts. Until now, my life has been just as it was predicted more than 3,000 years ago. As a result, I felt happy and relieved and longed even more for the adventure and experiences of the future. Figuratively, my reaction can be described as follows:

When I know the name of my destination and know that I am sitting in the right train to get there, I feel safe and can use my energy to enjoy the beautiful scenery. This is a completely different experience than previously, when I used my energy to worry whether I had got on to the wrong train and where the train I was sitting in, was heading for.

According to the astrologer, my reaction was as expected, because that it is exactly what the writing on the palm leaves in the past is for – to be a help to us "people of the future" in our lives. For example, by confirming that we are right in our actions or just to inspire us to dare to believe in what we do and perhaps will do later. Being prepared for what will happen, enables us to deal with the coming events in the best possible way.

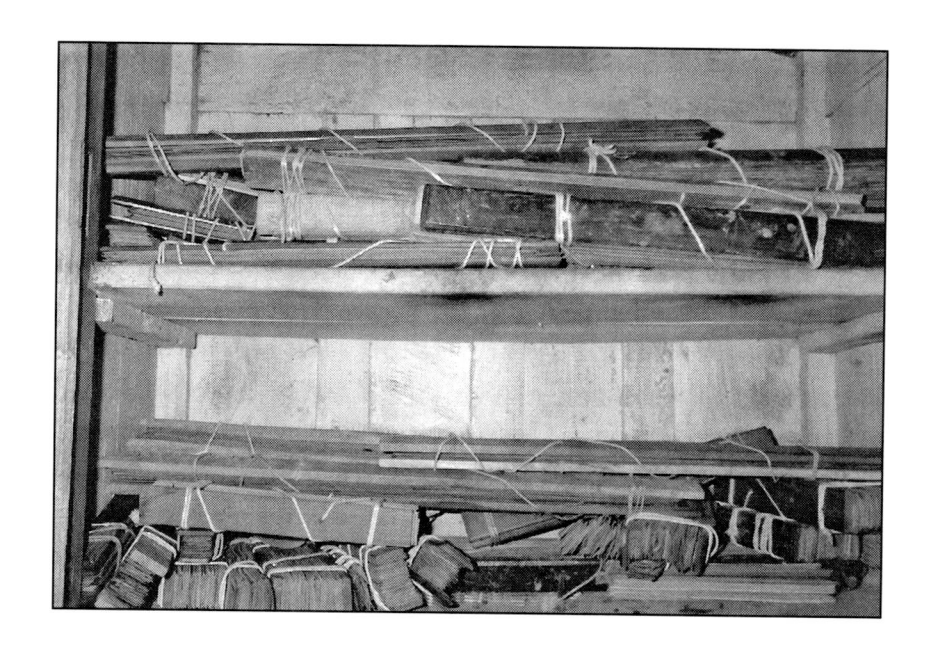

Palm leaf bundles filed on two shelves. See source information V

How the Palm Leaves call you

There is *not* a palm leaf for everyone in India. But the palm leaves that are in the archives will attract the right people at the right time. This may sound strange, and how it actually happens I cannot explain. But I will explain how I first came to hear about this palm leaf archive.

I was travelling with the Indian guru, Swamiji, about 800 km further up along the east coast of India. To be given the opportunity to be a part of this very interest group of travellers, was in itself a gift. I was one of four foreigners who were allowed to accompany him on his tour. In a small, poor town, we four foreigners were installed with an Indian family who were fond of the guru. On the last day the neighbour invited us for breakfast. The others accepted, but I was not interested. I wanted to wash some clothes and pack. When I was in the middle of washing clothes, the neighbour's wife came in. "We're waiting for you! Hurry up, come on!" she said. I could not ignore this invitation, so I put the clothes aside and went in to take part in the meal. Her husband was the town doctor and he had nothing at all to do with Swamiji. But he was interested in why four foreigners like us were travelling around with this guru. I told him that the reason I had come to India was to meet various gurus and palm leaf astrologers. That prompted him to tell us about his own experiences. He personally believed mostly in science and truths that can be measured and weighed. Even so, he had visited an astrologer who had been recommended by a friend. As he was explaining about this visit, I became interested. Particularly, because he only had to give his thumb print. Because of my obvious interest, the neighbour found an advertisement for the astrologer in which there were instructions on how to get there. I did not intend to visit that area during my journey, but kept the piece of paper just in case. Strangely enough, I was the only one of us four foreigners who was interested in having this piece of paper. It turned out later that the home of the palm leaf astrologer lay on the route I was travelling if I just made a small detour. Everything worked out for me, so this meeting could take place.

Is Palm Leaf Astrology a Con or a Fact?

The experiences with this special palm leaf astrologer, who found my palm leaf based on my thumb print, actually ended by extending the limits of my conceptual universe – I was shaken to the core. I still have not found a logical explanation as to how the astrologers there could know so much about me. But everything that was said about my past was true.

Later I also visited the palm leaf astrologer in New Delhi whose archives were based on information about time and place of birth. The information here at this astrologer's was on proper paper and thus copies of the original palm leaves. Although I gave him my birth data from the start, it took him a long time to find the "right piece of paper". It was not possible on my first visit – the information simply did not match the experiences I have had in my life. His explanation was that my time of birth was incorrect. I gave him more information about myself and on the basis of that he would look for my "correct" paper. It would take a few days, and therefore I had to come back again later. However, my subsequent meeting with him was interesting in some ways, because he also had information about me which I had not given and which would hardly match anyone else. But none of the information was of a kind that in any way enriched my life, and on "my paper", which did not contain any name, there was also some other information which I did not think matched mine. The whole atmosphere with this astrologer was oppressive and unconvincing. He also tried some worthless predictions. However, his attempt to get me to fall for his ploy was a little more elegant than what I had experienced with the astrologer in Chennai. His basis for demanding payment for prayers and rituals was that in this way I could help a sick relative. I do not care much for a palm leaf reading when the astrologer starts demanding large amounts of money to carry out special prayers. I would characterise that part of the séances as a con.

The method used by the astrologers to earn a lot of money from their clients is more or less the same with all of them. Therefore, I hope that the following description will prepare adventurous readers for the astrologers' tricks: By different routes they arrive at the fact that you have been the object of black magic. In time, such a blockage will poison your body, because it prevents the life energy from circulating freely. If you find it improbable that anyone should have laid a curse on you, they just say that it happened in a former life. Naturally, they are able to remove such blockages with some of their rituals and prayers in return for a suitable remuneration. You also have to carry a little container around your neck for the rest of your life, a talisman which contains various things from these rituals. If you yourself are fit and healthy and therefore difficult to get to take the bait, they try the other way round with your fellow human beings, as did the astrologer in New Delhi. As mentioned, he claimed that I could improve the condition of a sick relative by paying him to say prayers and rituals for this person. And who would not wish to help their nearest and dearest if it really could make a difference? Every time I was presented with such a story, I was shocked and angry, because they are clever at manipulating people. So if an astrologer does not allow the séance to be recorded, or if he turns the tape recorder off during the séance, there is a serious basis for suspicion. Because this happened during my first visit to an astrologer, I was very much on my guard with the subsequent astrologers, and I only felt comfortable and convinced with the special thumb print palm leaf astrologer.

But is up to oneself to assess what is a con and what is a fact. My experience that there was in India a palm leaf with the right name and data about my past indicates that in some way I am like a puppet. But whether everything is foretold, or whether we humans have our own free will? – Well ...

Information on prices and places

The price for visiting the palm leaf astrologer who used thumb prints was about 4.5 USD – 6.0 USD the appointment itself and 1.5 USD extra for an English translation of the content of the palm leaf written down in a notebook. The astrologer lives on the south-eastern coast of India, approximately 50 km north-west of the town of Nagapattinam. The address is:

Mr. A. Sivasamy, Nadi Astrologer
18, Milladi Street, Nagai District, Railway Station Road,
Opp. Indian Bank
Vaitheeswaran Koil – 609 117

Tamilnadu, SOUTH INDIA
Landline: +91-(0)4364-279463
Mobile: +91 9362227779 / +91 9489256905

http://srisivanadi.com/

[2017: I have updated the above information so that it applies to the present day. I have also added the home page address as it will contain the current data and also supplement with further information about this palm leaf astrologer and his work.]

I have since found out that there are other palm leaf astrologers in the same town who also use thumb prints as a basis. However, they have nothing to do with palm leaf archives described here. This astrologer disclaims any cooperation with them. There are no other departments or offices for these archives, neither in India nor abroad. Rumour has it that there is only a palm leaf for about 50 % of the people that come, and that the number is much smaller for Westerners.

With regard to price, the thumb print astrologer with the approximately 6 USD fee was much cheaper than the others. In comparison, I paid about 11 USD for the visit to the palm reader and astrologer in Chennai, and if I had fallen for his trick about black magic, it would have cost me 300-450 USD extra. The astrologer in New Delhi charged 100 USD as the basic rate. Furthermore, it cost another 50 USD if the time of birth I gave him was more than 10 minutes different from the time on the paper that matched me. Also here extra ceremonies against black magic cost an extra 300-450 USD. So my conclusion is that there is absolutely no correlation between price and quality.

As I mentioned previously, I had asked A. Sivasamy to forward more information from supplementary palm leaves. That cost about 6 USD extra. I paid the amount in complete confidence that I would soon hear from him. However, the information never arrived at the address in India which I had given. It was frustrating, because my disappointment cast a shadow over the otherwise positive visit with this astrologer. Therefore, I was very surprised and pleased when the answers arrived at my local post office six months later. The letter had been on a bit of a journey round India – in my wake – and had not caught up with me until here in Denmark.

Shree Maha Ganapathy Thunai,
Om Namo Narayanaya! Guruji Arumugam Kappu!!

☎ 79463
STD 04364

Sri Agasthiya Mahasiva Vakkiya
NADI JOTHIDA NILAYAM

A. SIVASAMY,
Nadi Astrologer,
S/o. V. S. ARULSIVA ARUMUGAM

| Don't be Misguided By Local Guides |

18, Milladi Street,
Vaitheeswarankoil-609 117
SIRKALI Tk.   Tanjore Dt.
Tamilnadu,   S. India.

Kandam No.   **LIST OF KANDAMS DETAILS**

1. To be found out through thumb impression (Gents Rights; Ladies Left) or horoscope of the concerned person Will contain name, parents names present details of profession, brothers sisters, children, wife and gist of future predictions for all the 12 houses.
2. Money, Eyes, Family, Education and speech.
3. Number of brothers and sisters, Affection, help or ill feeling in between self and brothers and sisters, Ears, Courage.
4. Mother, House, Vehicles, Lands and pleasures.
5. Children, Their Birth, reason for not having children, adoption of remedial measures for having children, future lives of the children.
6. Disease, Debts Enemies & Court Cases.
7. Time of marriage, Name, Lagnam, Planetary positions and distance of residence of the bride or bridegroom, Future life with husband or wife.
8. Longevity, Accident & Danger to Life. Age, Month, Date, Day, Time Star, Lagnam and Place of death.
9. Father-Prediction in regard to Father, Wealth Visit to temples. Luck, upadesam from holymen, charitable deeds.
10. Profession, Future predictions in regard to job or business, Change of place, good & evils in profession.
11. Profits and Second marriage.
12. Expenditure, Foreign Visit, Next birth & Attainment of salvation.
13. SANTHI PARIHARAM : Last birth. Sins committed, remedial measures for getting rid of the effect of the post birth's sins
14. DEEKSHAI KANDAM : Manthra jebam, Wearing of Rakshai (Talisman) for avoidance of enemies troubles etc.,
15. AUSHADHA KANDAM : Medicines for long standing disease and method of taking them
16. DISABUKTHI KANDAM : Predictions for the running Disa Bukthi (Major Sub. Period)

Note : i) Kandams 2 to 12 will give the future predictions up to the end of life from the date of perusal of that kandam.
ii) Special kandams viz **SIVANADI THULLIAM & SIVANADI SUKSHMAM** are also available Because of their specialised nature and elaborate details, fees will be higher. For success in **POLITICS** and **POLITICAL CONNECTIONS** special kandam is available. Other than the above kandams there are **Gnanakandam Prasna Kandam** and **Disabukthi Santhi Kandam.**
iii) Per day only two persons work can be attended.
iv) Should get prior date of appointment by post, Wednesday is holiday.
v) We do not have branches in any other place.
vi) Further Details Contact **BHAKKIAM LODGE.**
Phone Calls to 79463 will be attended between 8-30 a. m. to 6 p. m.

FOR A CONVENIENT STAY   **☎ 79460**
SHREE BHAKKIAM LODGE, South Car Street, Vaitheeswarankoil-609 117.

The front page of the advertisement for A. Sivasamy's Nadi Astrological Centre which I got from an Indian man on my journey. It explains which type of information the palm leaves contain

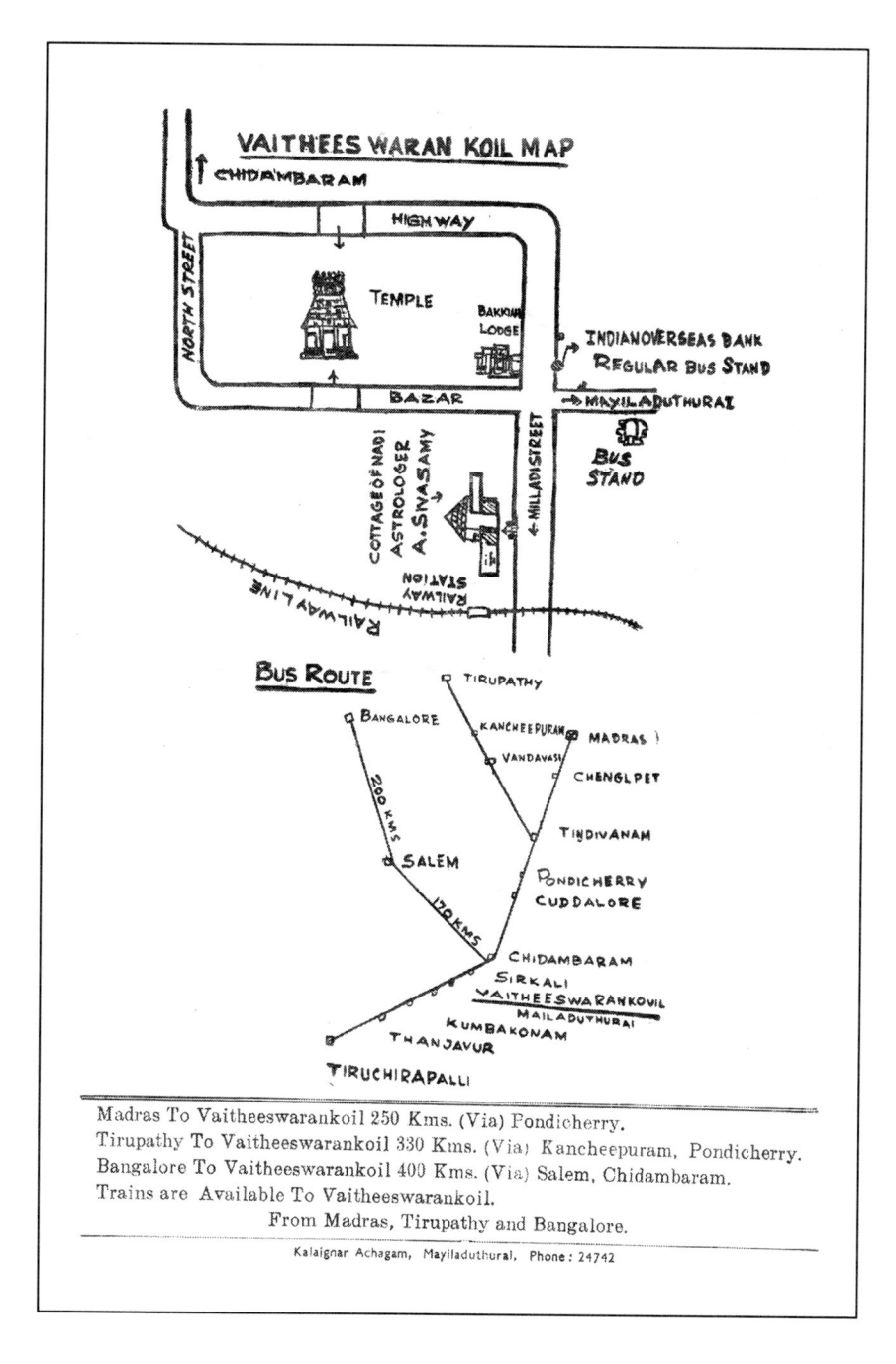

The back page of the advertisement for A. Sivasamy's Nadi Astrological Centre which I got from an Indian man on my journey. It shows a map of how to get there

INDIAN GURUS AND MY EXPERIENCES WITH THEM

What is a guru?

The word "guru" makes many westerners form the following image in their minds: a large, fat and very rich male person of Indian origin wearing orange robes. His followers flock around him like stupid sheep, because they have relinquished all responsibility and just direct their gaze at the guru in worship and ecstasy. The image usually has undertones of exploitation in the form of power, money or sex.

Admittedly, that was not the kind of image that made me travel to see the Indian gurus, but on the contrary my desire for knowledge and insight. And I was not the only one with this idea. I met people from all over the world when I was visiting the gurus. They were often highly educated people who were also deeply interested in the spiritual side of life.

The word "guru" is a combination of the words "gu", meaning "inner darkness" and "ru", meaning "he who destroys". The name indicates that the guru leads people from the darkness of ignorance to the light of wisdom. In India the word is used in many contexts in which it can be equated with the word "teacher". In the context of spiritual insight, the teaching matter of these gurus is just spiritual science instead of mathematics, for example.

The reason the term guru often has an almost divine overtone is because the "subject area" of the spiritual gurus is so intangible. For spiritual insight and wisdom belong in the borderland between what we feel, sense, experience and understand – and what we *believe*. And because belief is involved, there are all kinds of opportunities for manipulation. For anybody can call themselves guru, and there are many of them in India, both the bonafide ones and the fraudsters.

The Task of the True Gurus

The word "sad" means "truth" and a "Sadguru" is a guru whose task it is to show us the "truth" about ourselves. By "truth" is meant our own "divinity" which we can acknowledge by looking into our own hearts. Therefore, a Sadguru *never* assumes to be the Master, but helps us to see the Master in ourselves – our own Self – thereby helping us to attain the highest realisation. A quotation from the guru Swamiji describes the task of the Sadguru with the following image:

"God is within each one of us though it may not be possible for us to see him. The eyelids protect our eyes, and yet we cannot see them without the aid of a mirror. Similarly God is very much there, but we may not be able to see Him without the help of the Sadguru." (see source 25 on the first page)

My aim in visiting gurus

As mentioned in the preface, I have had an experience of the relativity of time. During this experience I found myself in a different and unknown state of consciousness. Therefore, I think it is probable that some people can have access to levels of consciousness with which other people are not normally in contact. Perhaps the gurus have an "aerial" which reaches higher up than mine so that they can receive signals which I normally cannot catch. Although the choice of gurus might perhaps be of varying quality, nevertheless I was not going to let it prevent me from seeking out the real thing: gurus from whom I could learn something. Before my departure I had selected four gurus that I wanted to visit:

Ganapati Sachchidananda Swamiji – also called Swamiji,
Sathya Narayana Raju – also called Sathya Sai Baba or Baba,
Mata Amritanandamayi – also called Amma or Divine Mother,
H.W.L. Poonja – also called Poonjaji or Papaji.

One may perhaps read the messages of the gurus in a book, but their charisma has to be felt in one's own body and soul. I felt attracted to the idea of an experience of this kind. I was aware beforehand that the teachings of these four gurus were not contrary to my own convictions. Apart from this basic knowledge, I was not interested in reading more about their methods. Instead I wished to have a personal meeting with them in order to experience and ascertain whether the gurus really were special, or whether they were just ordinary people who by chance had become the object of other people's adoration and love. It is known that at least two of them can materialise, that is to say create physical objects out of apparently thin air. I wanted to see this with my own eyes. By meeting them it was my aim to learn more about some of the mysteries of life: *Who are we as human beings?* and *Is there any limit to what is possible?*

Ashram: a home for gurus and their students

On the practical level, all four gurus are in daily contact with their students. I will take the liberty of also using the word *students* about the helpers, staff members and all the other people who spend some time close to the guru. For practical reasons the gurus often live and work in the same place – in their ashram – where many of the students also live. The word "ashram" means "cave", thus describing the place where gurus used to seek refuge in order to worship their god(s) away from the noise and bustle of the outside world. Today many gurus have replaced their caves with houses in and outside the towns. These places, where one can stay with the purpose of introspection and contemplation with the divine and spend time introspecting according to one's faith, are still called ashrams. The idea is to create a basis for rendering optimum spiritual service. The ashrams of the true Masters are charged with the high spiritual vibration of the gurus, thus contributing to the transformation of the students. Some ashrams just consist of a single house, while others are whole towns. For example, many thousands of students can stay at Sai Baba's ashram in Puttaparthi, which besides a temple also contains apartment blocks, restaurants, shops and small factories. Many gurus also have several ashrams spread around India and abroad. By travelling around to these ashrams, the gurus reach out to a larger group of people who in this way have their local place where they can gather with others to practice their faith. In order to get the most out of my visits to the gurus, I had planned to stay in their ashrams as far as possible.

My attitude to life and "God"

Naturally, my experiences with the gurus must be seen in the light of my own personal attitude to life. Therefore, I will start by explaining my stance.

For me the concept of God covers EVERYTHING. To me God is not an object and is therefore without form. Any attempt at a description would be a limitation of the "Infinite Universe" and thus not be a description of it. I use the word God for The Highest One, who may be given different names in different religions, but who ultimately must be The One and Only. Instead of the word "God", I might tentatively use concepts such as the omnipresent and all-pervading love, intelligence, vibration, wisdom and truth. When I use the word "divine" in the following, I am therefore referring to these qualities.

I find it natural to observe life from the principle of reincarnation, that is to say that we humans are reborn several times on the earth. With every earth life we come across circumstances which enable us to attain wisdom through experience. The aim is finally to be able to acknowledge our true nature and unity with God. Then we will have finished our task here on earth and can continue to live in other dimensions or universes. This conviction is not connected to any specific religion, and I do not perceive some people as being more divine than others; we are all a part of the divine whole. But I do believe that some people have progressed further in the process of acknowledgement concerning our true origins and that they have greater insight and experience. In this they have attained a higher spiritual level and their level of vibration has been increased. It is in the light of this that the gurus come into the picture – both as far as I and other spiritual seekers are concerned. I was not ready to allow any of them to change my attitude to life, but if they really have acknowledged their true nature and themselves achieved becoming one with the divine vibration, perhaps they might be able to teach me more about myself, other people, life, the universe, the whole and – not least – love.

My reactions to the presence of the gurus

At the first meetings with the four gurus, it soon became clear to me that they all exerted a completely peculiar attraction. The air vibrated in a strange way around them. It was my heart in particular that was touched by their presence. They radiated love much more intensely than ordinary people. It was as if invisible nectar flowed from them for which my body and soul hungered and lapped up. The more I got, the more I wanted.

The four gurus each have their own way of working in their daily routines. Some carry out Hindu rituals, while others do not wish to use rituals. In order to get the most out of my visits, I decided to participate in all the official events with each guru. This also meant that the daily rhythm was somewhat different than in Denmark. You normally get up very early in the ashrams, and it is actually rather nice to enjoy the cool morning hours before the heat of the sun lays its blanket of drowsiness over everything. But whatever ceremonies the gurus might stage on the outer level, they all work on the inner level with the people present. At least, that is my explanation for what happened. For each guru produced the same patterns of reaction in me.

I did not understand the context of things with my mind, but emotionally I felt different than usual. Old suppressed feelings came up to the surface without any immediate reason. In contact with a guru most people do not avoid a good cry – and neither did I. It just happens, whether or not you are used to crying or normally never show tears. One of the sharpest and fastest reactions was the tiredness which quickly overpowered me. I could not do without my afternoon nap; sometimes I slept up to several hours in the middle of the day. There can also be physical changes such as fever, diarrhoea, inflammation, pain and many other effects. In particular, I suffered from fever and headaches, but it varies individually depending on the weak points of the body. It was my impression that just being physically near a guru puts you automatically through the physical and mental wringer. Naturally, this can be very unpleasant while it is happening. But afterwards it is a great relief when heavy burdens from your baggage have been cast away. For me, part of this "cleansing" was about taking stock and clearing up. Either by writing letters and saying to others what had never been said, or by just creating closure for things in my own heart. It is difficult to explain what actually goes on during this process. You just have to let things go their own way and try to make the best of the situation. The result can be clearly seen in the eyes afterwards; there is much more life, light, joy, warmth and clarity.

A possible explanation for their influence

The following image can illustrate how I perceive the exchange that occurs when I am close to a guru: if – using a rough comparison – a person is equated with a pan filled with water, if you compare a person to a pan filled with water; the content is the same whether or not the water is boiling or cold. The only difference is the speed at which each individual water molecule is moving. The faster it moves around, the hotter the water gets. Although the substance of the guru and myself is the same – like the water – the guru's is hotter than mine, because he has access to more energy. When my pan gets close to the guru's, which might even be boiling, the heat from this will affect and heat up my water. Before there might even have been ice on the surface of my water. The meeting then causes this ice structure to be broken up and dissolved. If I have been used to identifying myself by virtue of this ice crust, I might at first start to panic, for who am I if it no longer exists? Although I am the same pan of water as I always have been, it is my experience of myself that must change. I must look at myself in a new way in order to accept my new shape without the ice crust. When the ice breaks up, some impurities will automatically be released in the body and mind. They come up to the surface and then disappear. The mind is cleansed, in among other ways, by tears – the body uses the channels which are available. The result is that when the surface is no longer covered by ice, the water has much greater freedom of movement. This is why I was not aware that they existed within my framework – and maybe there is no framework or limitations as to who and how we are as human beings ...

General remarks about the messages of the four gurus

My choice of precisely the four gurus mentioned was mainly based on friends having warmly recommended them. Papaji was the only one that I had met before on my previous journey to India. When I left to go on this new journey, I still did not possess any special knowledge about the religion and culture of the country or the other three gurus. I was just filled with curiosity and the desire for exciting experiences. I had, however, heard enough about the gurus to know that we had the same basic attitude. And of course, a common reference is the best basis for a fruitful cooperation. The common characteristics of the four gurus are:

- that they do not profess to any religion, but only to the highest truth,
- that they are Sadgurus, i.e. they will try to teach us to find and rest in our own inner true being – our divine nature,
- that humanity works as the predominant part of their nature, and
- that it is free to participate in their ceremonies and listen to their speeches

The fundamental basis for these four gurus is the Vedanta philosophy: that we are all a part of the same divine whole. What they wish to show us can be expressed in one Sanskrit word: *sat-chit-ananda*. This word can be translated to *divine-existence-(and)knowledge* and therefore *knowledge of divine existence*, as "sat" means "existence", "chit" means "knowledge" and "ananda" means "divinity". If we have lost contact with this essence, it is simply because we ourselves have directed our awareness in other directions.

The gurus' task is, therefore, to show their students the path back to their true inner identity, in among other ways by pointing out that feelings, thoughts and our daily dramas are not our true source. In the same way that many roads lead to Rome, there are many paths to realisation, and these four gurus each have their own methods for leading their students on to the right path. It is just up to each individual to choose the path they find most attractive, if they desire at all to try out any of the gurus' guidelines, methods and tools. I did. In fact I hungered to both smell and taste the special dish of each guru in order to see whether there were any which suited me.

My experiences with and impressions of each guru

When I met a guru for the first time and tried to form an impression of him, I tended to observe and assess every little thing that went on. It was rather exhausting. However, in time I learnt to disregard the outer actions and instead moved my attention to the important thing: my heart's contact with the guru. This heart contact is difficult to describe with words. I experienced it as a vibration of energy around my heart, almost as if I had a string in my heart which had been made to vibrate. The vibration touched something deep and filled my body with peace and wellbeing. It was not until this heart contact was established that I could begin to understand the meaning of the gurus' daily rituals and routines. It transpired each time that when I understood the symbolism in these ritual actions, my experiences of them intensified.

Swamiji

My meeting with Swamiji was not a sudden revelation. But little by little I got to know him, and the more I learned the more astonished and fascinated I became. At that time he was a handsome Indian man of 52 years (born 1942). He had wonderful deep and caring eyes which made me wish to always gaze into them. He was spontaneously mild and friendly in manner and radiated caring and tenderness. It felt as if he was both a divine mother and father rolled into one, and in fact a child also. A kind of non-gender being or rather perhaps an all-gender being.

I knew nothing about Swamiji when I left for India, but a good friend had recommended visiting this guru. A visit with him was my first goal on my trip. I travelled straight from Copenhagen, Denmark, to the town of Vijayawada in Western India, where Swamiji was staying. I knew that he would only be at this place for another four days. Swamiji's main ashram is in the town of Mysore south of Bangalore, but at that time he was touring the other local ashrams in Southern India. I arrived at the ashram at seven in the evening after travelling for 33 hours. I was fairly tired, but still proud to have succeeded in finding this precise house in this gigantic country. In the ashram, the guru and his followers were singing and playing music together. Swamiji was giving talks between the numbers which he played on his synthesizer accompanied by violins and drums. The event was taking place in the yard in front of the house. Several hundred Indians were sitting on the flagstones, singing along or listening. At the entrance gate, where I was standing among the sandals of the people in the audience, a person who looked like a staff member spoke to me. I gave him the name of a friend of a friend whom I did not know myself, but who I knew would be there. After a while this man came and took me with him to the queue. For now the audience had started to queue up to give Swamiji money belts. These could be bought for a few pennies and given to the guru as a sign of affection. I bought some too as a greeting to this guru. When I gave him them, Swamiji smiled at me. My new friend told me that it was a good sign.

Next on the agenda was to find a place to sleep. This ashram consisted of only one block of buildings with very few sleeping quarters. The Indians slept in the yard or in the dining room wrapped in their blankets. My friend's friend was the only one who had his own room.

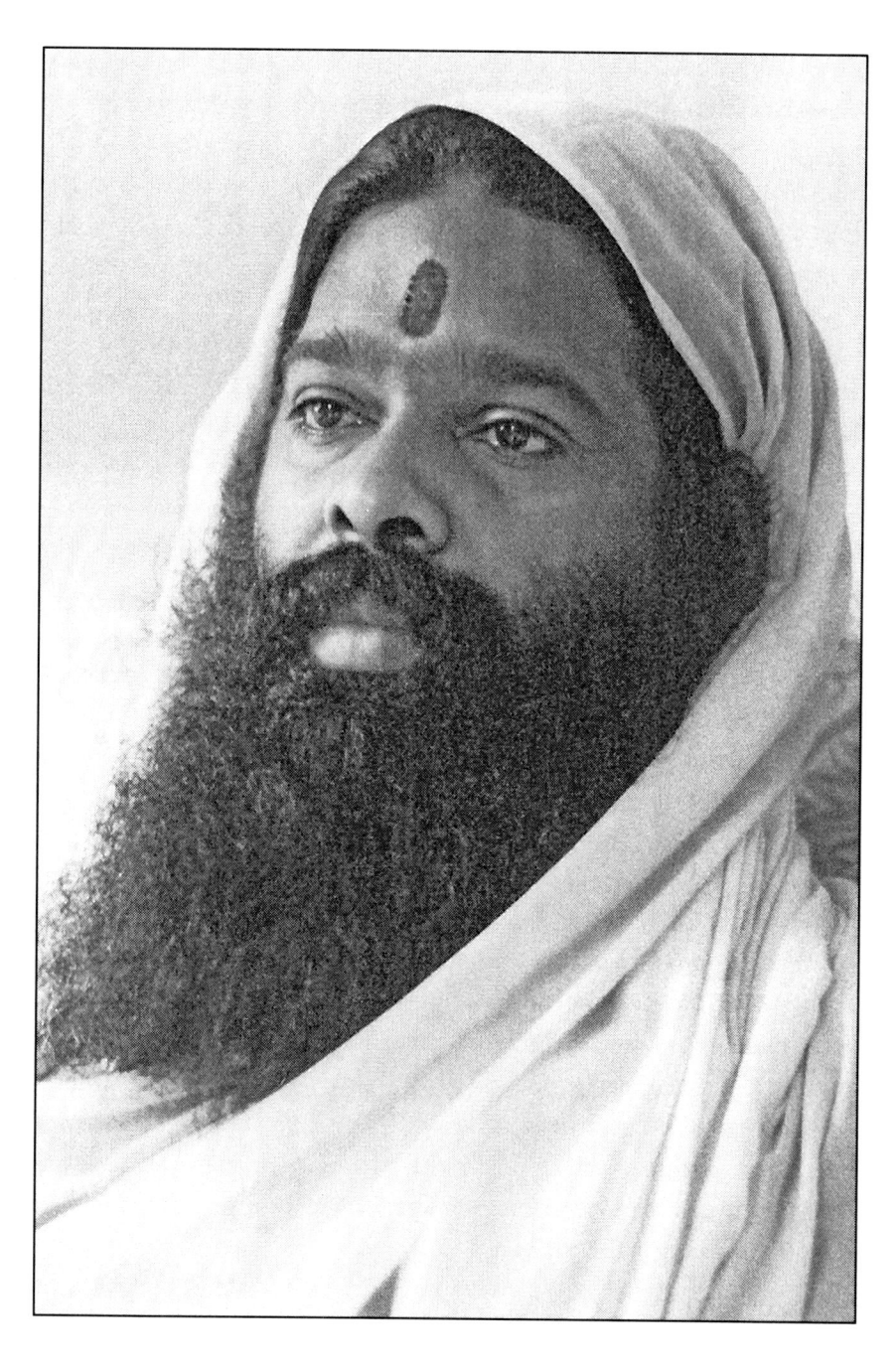

Sri Ganapati Sachchidananda Swamiji. See source information VI

After long consideration, he decided that I could sleep on the floor outside his tent which was pitched in the room to serve as a mosquito net. I felt very privileged and happy that I did not have to go to a hotel, but instead could stay so close to Swamiji. He was going to stay another four days in this ashram, after which he would continue on his tour. I wanted to make the most of my short time with him.

In this ashram the bathroom facility was a raw concrete room of only 1½ m² containing a cold water tap at hip level, a bucket and a dipper. We were ten foreigners who had to bathe at least twice a day in this room. The lavatories were stinking squat toilets with no toilet paper, but with a tap on the left side which is how they clean themselves in most of India. What was strange and surprising for me was the fact that even though I had arrived the same evening straight from Denmark, did not know a single soul, slept on a dirty stone floor and was bitten all over by mosquitoes, I had a strong sensation of having come home. During my previous trip to India I had never had this feeling, nor in any other places than in Denmark where I live. But in some inexplicable way, this was apparently also my home. On an inner level it felt familiar, loving, pleasant and safe to be near Swamiji and the people that surrounded him.

The other approximately 20 foreigners who had also come to this place with Swamiji, were very kind and pleasant, and I immediately felt at ease among them. Swamiji carried out some ceremonies every day, and the first day I watched them and him. During the communal singing on this first evening, I submitted with dignity to being bored and I endured my seat on the floor for the two hours it took. But already on the second day I began to be aware at the morning ceremony of how much energy was activated in the room before Swamiji arrived, while specially chosen people were sitting chanting their prayers. I had no previous experience or knowledge of mantras which, as previously mentioned, are prayers which are repeated over and over in the sacred language Sanskrit. Neither could I imagine that they could be particularly special. But my experience in the crowd of people aroused my curiosity for I felt an impact from this song inside my body where I sensed a special vibration. Of course, the energy intensified even more when Swamiji finally joined us.

The following afternoon I seized the opportunity to take part in a ceremony in which every person was allowed to ask Swamiji a few questions. I was rather disappointed that he could not promise me that I would meet the prince on a white steed later in life and that we would have children. He either would or could not confirm my dreams for the near future. Instead Swamiji said that I should learn about Hinduism and the like, which did not please me at all. The other foreigners saw my disappointment and heard the answers I was given. I concluded that perhaps this guru was not so interesting after all, because my primary goal in this life was a loving family life.

Later in the day, a German man approached me. He had heard about the answers I had received from Swamiji. The German told me that he had been studying spiritual philosophy and various religions for many years and he had an overview which I would not be able to find in any book. Furthermore, he had a structured method of working and if I was interested, he would give me lessons. In spite of my disappointment I did not want to reject such an offer and in the course of the next few days my ears developed to "elephant size". It turned out that this man had the overview which made all the pieces in my puzzle fall into place. I understood the origin of every religion and the basis of the guru's work. It was as if all my knowledge was gathered together to form a whole. Suddenly there was a natural connection between my outlook on life and my interest for spirituality and this strange religion: Hinduism. At the same time, I began to experience the evening song and music events as enjoyable instead of boring, and I started to regard this Swamiji with curiosity again.

The three ceremonies which Swamiji performed every day are called pooja, homa and bhajan. During the *pooja* he cleaned a small figure "Sri Chakra", which symbolises the universe and the universal energy.

During the *homa* he offered special fruits, flowers etc. to the fire while the people present could send their wishes and prayers with them out into the universe. Both these ceremonies took place in the morning. In the afternoon there was *bhajan*. This is communal singing and music in which the lyrics praise the gods and love. During these séances, Swamiji sometimes held talks in the local Indian language, telegu. Fragments were only rarely translated from Indian to English and they were not always comprehensible for a Dane like me. Swamiji was mostly surrounded by specially chosen people and close staff members who joined in the reciting of the mantras and generally helped while he performed the daily rituals. As I only understood a little of what was said and almost nothing of the ceremonies, I was forced to just feel how it was for me to sit among the audience and experience what was going on. There were English books about Swamiji and his speeches on sale at the ashram. But, as mentioned, I preferred to experience rather than read. Swamiji himself declares that his main objective is to heal people through music. For music has a quality which penetrates and does something to our minds and bodies without our thoughts being able to control and understand what is happening. The music arrangements made room for many musicians who were all given the opportunity and space to show their skills, because each number had a basic melody on which they could improvise. Swamiji guided the course of the arrangements at the same time as playing his synthesiser, and often he also sang. He was always accompanied by at least two kinds of drums – tablas – and one violin, but the band could be expanded by more of these instruments or other kinds such as other drums, flutes etc. Swamiji regularly holds large concerts all over India at which the best known musicians of the country play with him. Although many of these normally are competitors, they will make an exception and cooperate on these occasions. None of them want to miss out on taking part at his performance.

The first three days I spent with Swamiji passed quickly and he was about to move on. Only three foreigners who had a special function to perform were allowed to accompany him. I wanted most of all to go with him and when I saw an opportunity to ask Swamiji for permission

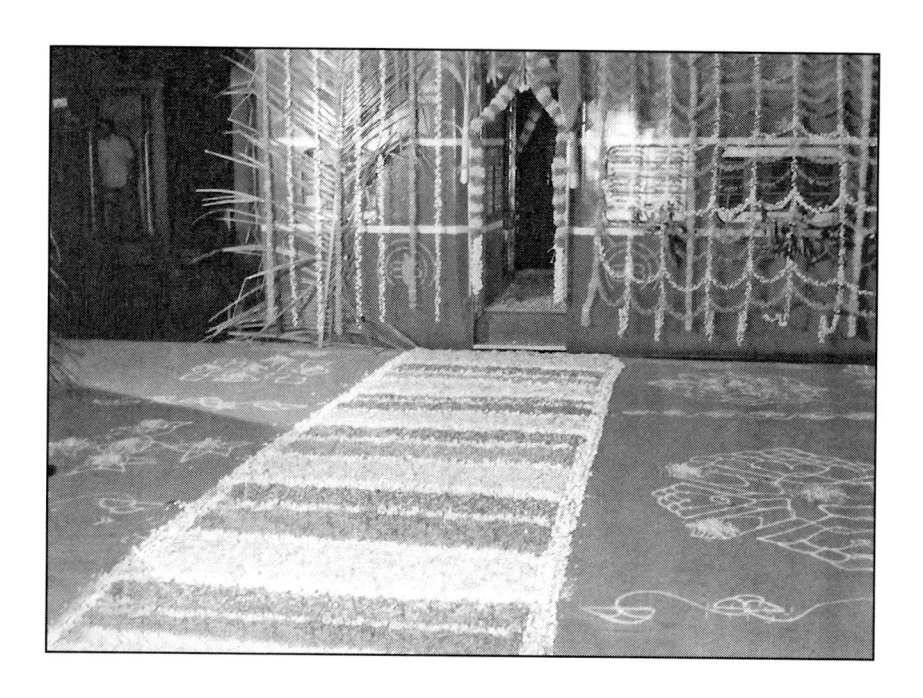

The train carriage for Swamiji's journey was decorated inside and out with flowers. Photo: Lisbeth Ejlertsen

directly, he said yes. Everyone was surprised at this and some were even angry. For I had only known this guru for three days and others had known him for many years. But I was happy and enjoyed the following nine days where I had the great experience and pleasure of accompanying Swamiji on his journey. It consisted of visits to various ashrams and private homes as well as participation in various music events and concerts which Swamiji gave. I often had the thought that Swamiji's reception in the various towns might be compared to the entry of Jesus into Jerusalem. Because everywhere there were hundreds of people to welcome him, and everything was decorated with fresh flowers, including cars, trains, buildings and the special welcome arches which were built for him. Even at the stations where Swamiji's train only stopped for a few minutes, the platforms were decorated and crowded with people who wanted to express their devotion.

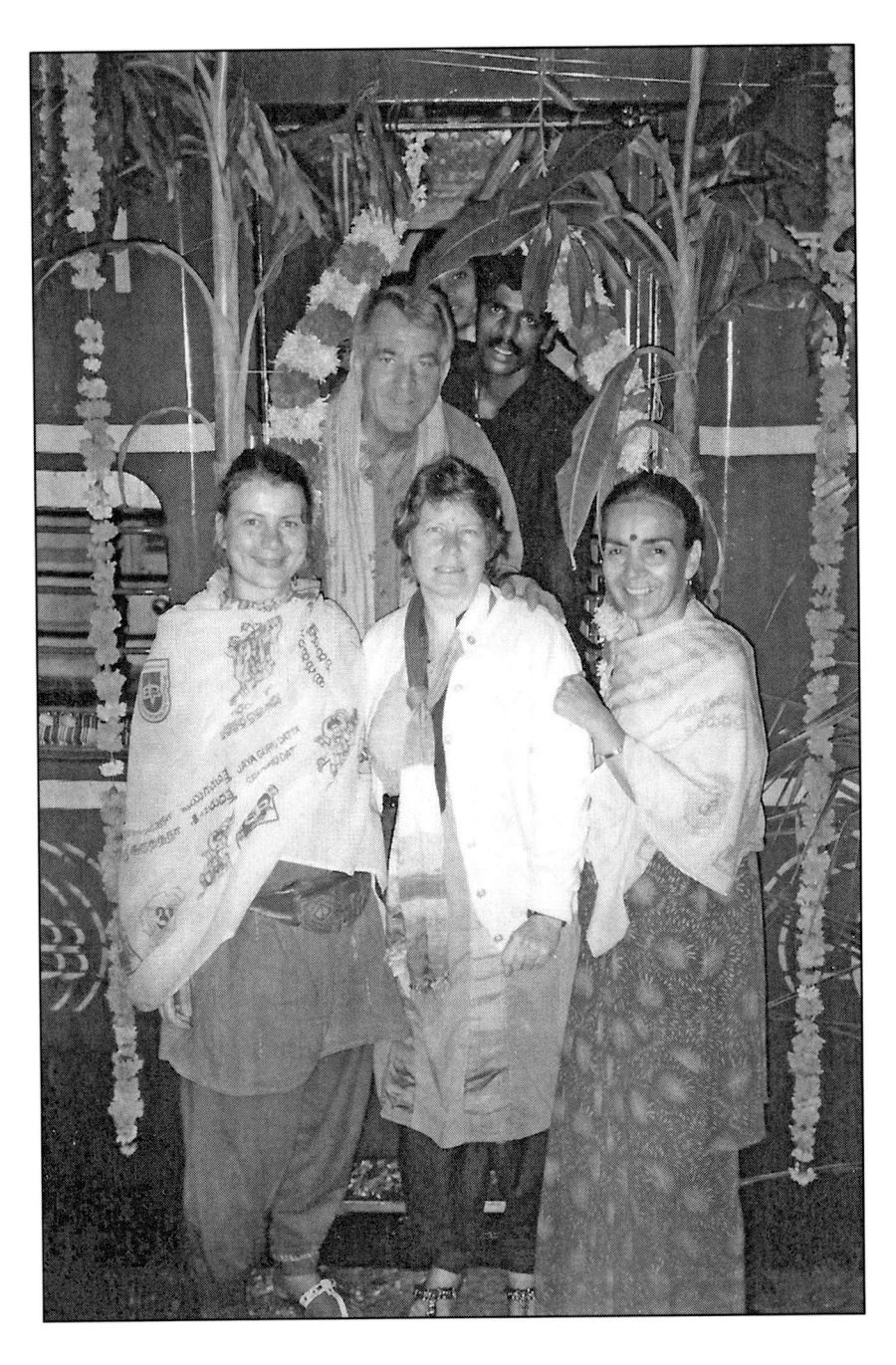

We four foreigners who accompanied Swamiji on a part of his journey. Photo: Unknown person who was present

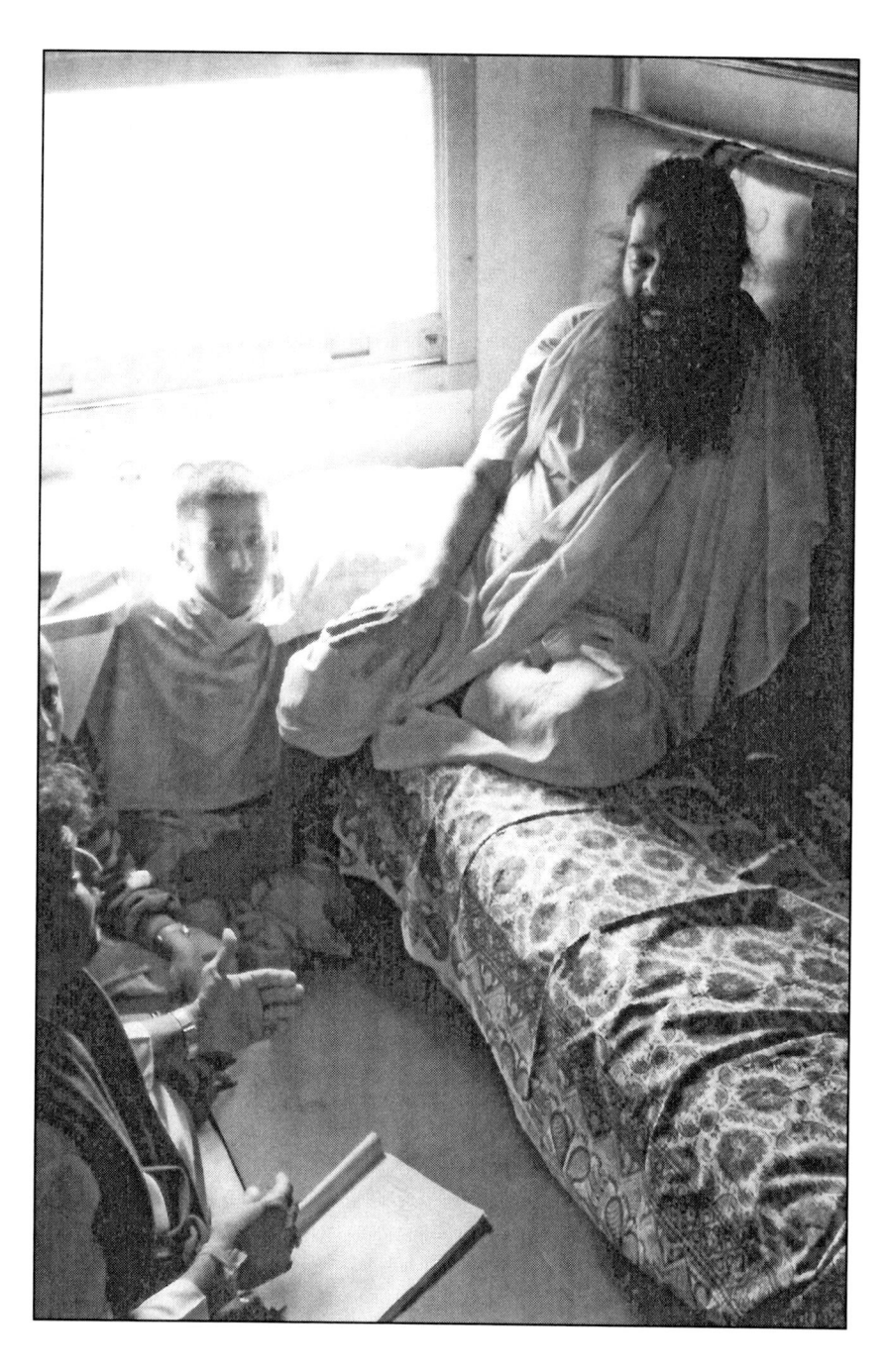

*A quiet moment on the train journey with Swamiji
and his entourage. Photo: Lisbeth Ejlertsen*

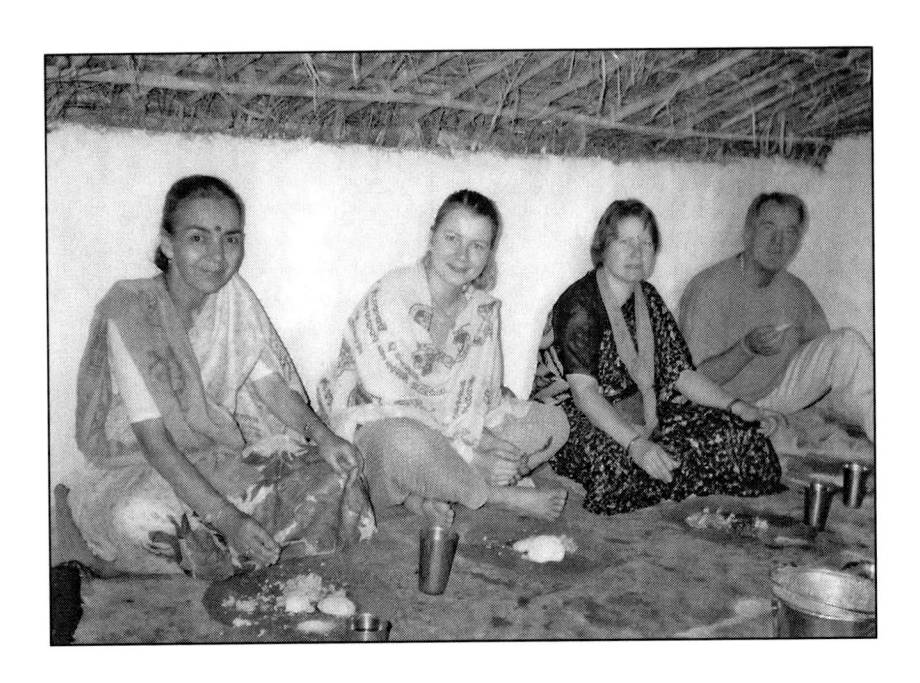

Lunching in the Indian manner in one of Swamiji's smaller and simpler ashrams. Photo: Unknown person who was present

Other foreigners who had known Swamiji for several years could relate many fascinating stories which I was happy to listen to. I personally had the following experience which made me wonder what kind of person Swamiji really was. When I had known him only three days and while we still were in the ashram at Vijayawada, I felt a desire to ask him for an Indian name. It often happens that a guru gives his students a new name as an exercise in how to take a new look at oneself. But for me it was just an idea that I initially kept to myself. Later that day, one of Swamiji's staff members had to note down the names and ages of us four foreigners who were to accompany him on the trip. The others stated their names. Instead of asking for my name, the Indian just wrote down the name of an Indian goddess. I asked why and was told that this goddess' name matched the Indian god name which one of the other foreigners had been given. According to their stories of the gods, this goddess was a travelling companion to the god whose name he carried. I let this Indian do as he wanted and thought no more about

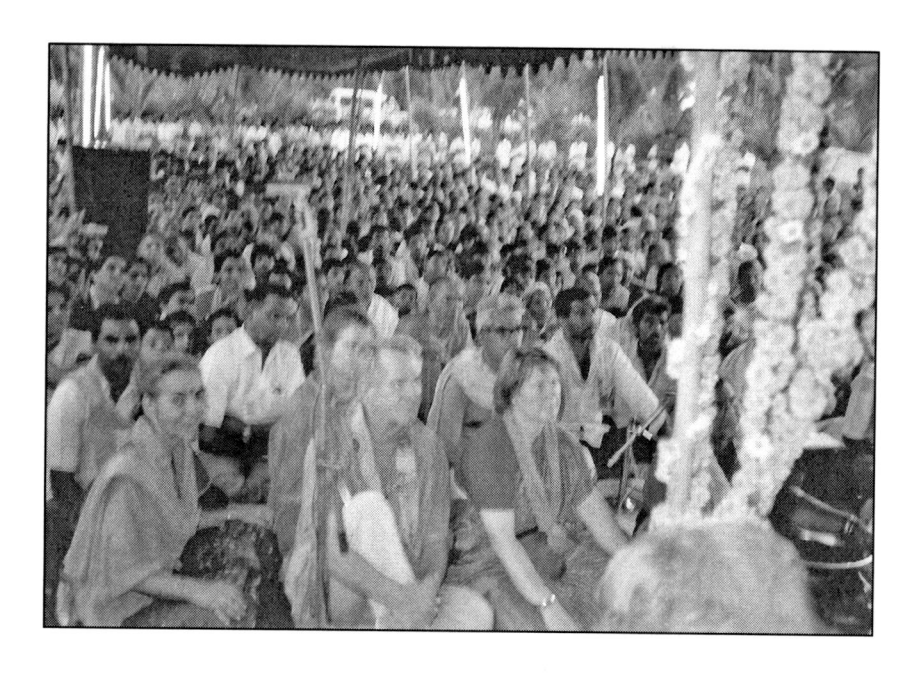

At every stop we made on the journey many people had turned up to meet Swamiji. Photo: Unknown person who was present

it until a couple of days later during our train journey when I gave Swamiji a letter. At this point – to my own surprise – I took a new and completely unforeseen step: in the letter I asked Swamiji to give me a new name. Later he came into our compartment and asked the other foreigners what he should call me. They had been present at the above mentioned episode with the ticket seller, so one of them mentioned with a laugh the name the ticket seller had given me. Swamiji nodded and then allotted that name to me. This all seemed quite coincidental to me, but about one month later, when I was in a completely different place in India with the palm leaf astrologer, he read out just this same Indian name from a palm leaf on which my Danish name was also written. As mentioned, the information on the palm leaf was more than 3,000 years old. So Swamiji had given me the name that I was predestined to have. And that was not all. He had given me the name via his staff member before I had actually asked for it, because at that point I had only thought to ask for an Indian name in my own thoughts which expressed themselves in my own language, Danish!

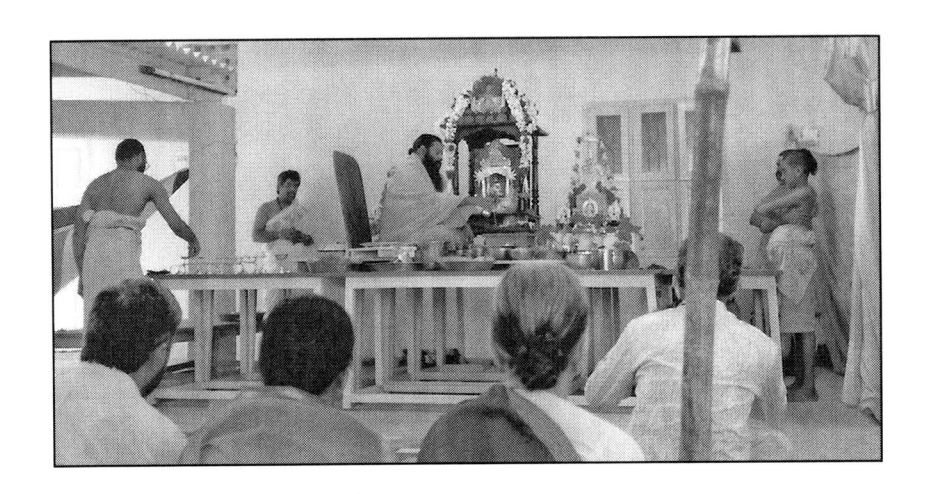

Every morning, also during the journey, Swamiji carries out a pooja ceremony. Photo: Lisbeth Ejlertsen

Swamiji can also materialise objects and does it regularly to catch people' attention. But what he basically has to offer to people is friendship in the sense that he can give you support to develop yourself. If life is about human beings developing through the experiences they harvest, then it is no good if Swamiji removes all suffering by a miracle. For suffering animates us to learn to deal with problems and is thus the portal to greater capaciousness and understanding of ourselves and our fellow human beings. Through friendship with Swamiji the learning process is made shorter and easier. His followers can be found both among the poorest and the richest, and also include civil servants and ministers. Besides several ashrams in India, Swamiji also has centres in the US and France.

I cannot explain specifically why or how Swamiji moved so deeply into my heart and opened doors to chambers there which had never been open before. Sometimes the tears ran down my cheeks for no other reason than the sensation of being part of an all-embracing love. On the rest of my journey round India, I returned to him several times.

Sai Baba

Sai Baba is probably the best known of these four gurus and at this point in time he was 68 years old (born 1926). His charisma felt very powerful and his physical body seemed almost ethereal. A feeling of deep calm and relaxation spread through my body whenever he passed by.

Many people have a sensation that Sai Baba is practically asking them to come to his ashram. They say that he has contacted them in dreams and called them to him in this way. Nothing like that had happened to me; I just arrived without this kind of special invitation.

Being in his ashram Puttaparthi was a special experience, because it is in fact a whole town. It was clean and well organised everywhere. For example, the ashram had its own water supply and it was quite a relief to be able to brush one's teeth and take a shower without worrying about swallowing polluted water at the same time. Also the food, which could be bought at the ashram, was safe to eat; it was clean and nourishing.

Sai Baba's daily contact with people took place when he appeared four times a day at the ashram's temple square. During the six days I spent there about 7-10,000 people gathered in the temple square each time to attend Sai Baba's ceremonies. Two of the four times Sai Baba received letters "darshan" and the other two times there was singing, "bhajan". During these ceremonies most people had to be content to see him pass by quite a long way off. The only opportunity to get close to Sai Baba was to get to sit in one of the rows at the front and thus closest to Sai Baba when he came into the temple square. Every time Sai Baba was coming we were all gathered in a special area and herded into many queues where we had to stand in line. The principle of "chance" reigned when the queues were finally given numbers – that is if you believe in chance. The current number decided how soon your queue was allowed to go into the temple square. You were lucky if you were in the chosen queue which was allowed to go first. The later your queue was chosen, the further back on the square you would be sitting.

However, there was another small chance to meet Sai Baba – a meeting of a more private nature. Every day he also gave "interviews" to about 20-30 people. Although they were called interviews, they resembled more meetings in the precise sense of the word "meetings". To get such an interview you had either to sit in one of the foremost lines so that you could hand a letter to Sai Baba and ask for an interview there, or you could be in a group with someone who got an interview. If just one person from a group was sitting in the front row and was given permission for an interview, the rest of the group was automatically included. Therefore the visitors often divided up into groups of about 10-20 people in order to increase their chances of a closer contact to Sai Baba. During my stay I took part every day in all four ceremonies and before each ceremony I joined a group. Even so I saw Sai Baba about five minutes at the most at each ceremony and never got to attend an interview.

Sai Baba is very eager to support the Indian people through help to self-help. He takes care of the whole town around the ashram, partly by employing many of inhabitants in his ashram, and partly by building houses and schools for them. He has built universities, a hospital, a water supply plant, a museum and a planetarium in the area. They are all equipped according to the best western standards.

In spite of these good acts, he also has enemies. About two years ago there was an attempted assassination against Sai Baba. Therefore, all visitors have to go through a metal detector at the entrances to the temple square before each ceremony. With the great number of visitors, this meant a lot of waiting around. The assistants, who were supposed to keep order and assign places to the visitors in the temple square before the daily rituals, behaved in a surly and unfriendly manner, to put it mildly. It sometimes felt rather provocative to be pushed around from one queue to another and more or less to be forced to sit on the laps of the other visitors in the mercilessly baking heat of the sun. Men and women were sharply divided in the ashram. This applied to the sleeping quarters, the restaurants and the temple square. Even if you

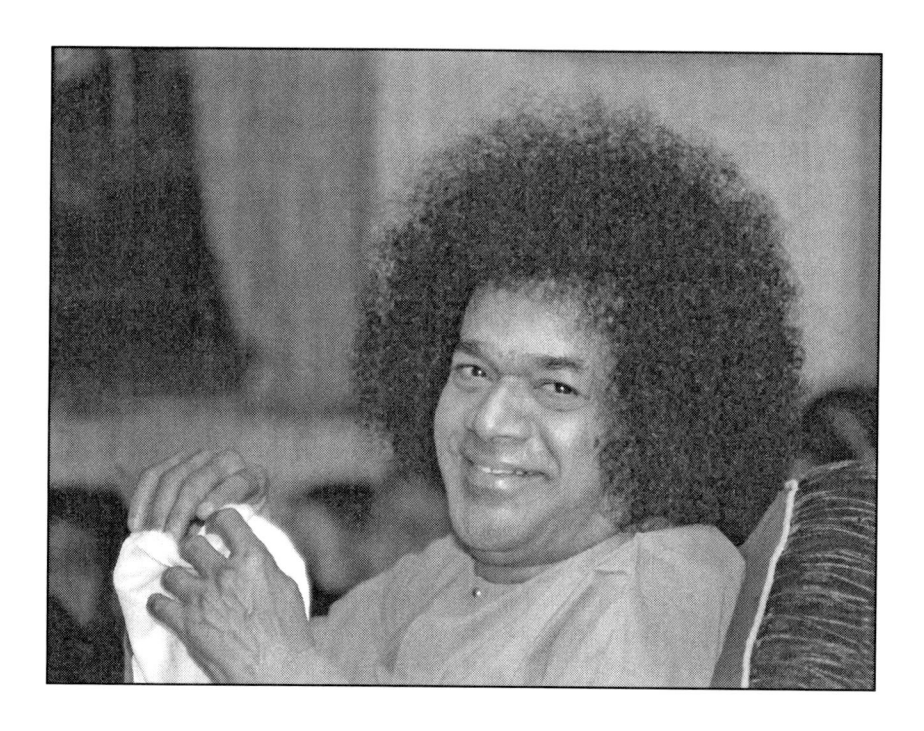

Satya Sai Baba. Photo: See source information VII

stood talking to someone of the opposite sex on the ordinary roads in the ashrams, the guards would come and disperse the group. For a westerner like me it was a little difficult to understand the meaning of these strict rules. However, my resistance to some of the outer things did not prevent me from experiencing all the other things which were nice and pleasant.

One of the things I loved doing during my stay there was cracking coconuts in front of a large statue of the elephant god, Ganapati. This was a very physical act, because you needed to use your strength to crack the hard shells on the coconuts, but at the same time it could also have a very fine symbolic value. For the shell is regarded as being an image of the human ego: the part of us which acts out of vanity and hunger for power. Contrary to this, the juicy meat and the coconut milk reflect our inner softness and treasures – the love behind the facade. When a nut has been cracked in front of Ganapati, half is thrown in to the god figure and the rest is shared with the people standing around. In this way you show your desire to strip away your ego and afterwards your desire to share your inner values with God and people. For those who regard Ganapati as a representative of the divine in ourselves, the act symbolises an attempt at inner transformation: from self-centred to a more open and sensitive being.

I was a little disappointed that I did not get close to Sai Baba during the visit. He can also materialise objects, and I would have liked to have seen that close up. But as only about 20-30 people a day were given the opportunity for a meeting, it was not very probable that I would be among the lucky ones. In the course of my six day stay at the ashram, I got used to the conditions and ended by enjoying it. I was deeply touched by meeting Sai Baba and yet not at all unhappy to leave there. Perhaps it was because my inner self was still full of the experiences with Swamiji.

Amma

"Amma" is an Indian word for "mother". The name suits this guru woman perfectly, because I experienced Amma as the epitome of the archetypal mother figure. At that point in time she was 41 years old (born 1953) and she had a gentle and caring nature. I would compare her energy to that of the moon. It does not shine directly in your eyes, but nonetheless it is very forceful in its own deep way. Twice a week Amma held a special form of "darshan". On these occasions people flocked to her ashram from far and near, and she often sat up to eight hours without a break and shared out one hug after another. She would give several thousand hugs at one session. She poured out her love on everyone by hugging every single person and whispering incomprehensible words in their ears. It was her way of blessing people and everyone was always welcome to her blessing – her darshan. There was also daily bhajan at the ashram. This communal singing, which I seldom experience in Denmark, became a welcome part of my daily life in India. It was lovely and peaceful to sit with the others during the communal singing, even though I did not understand any of the lyrics.

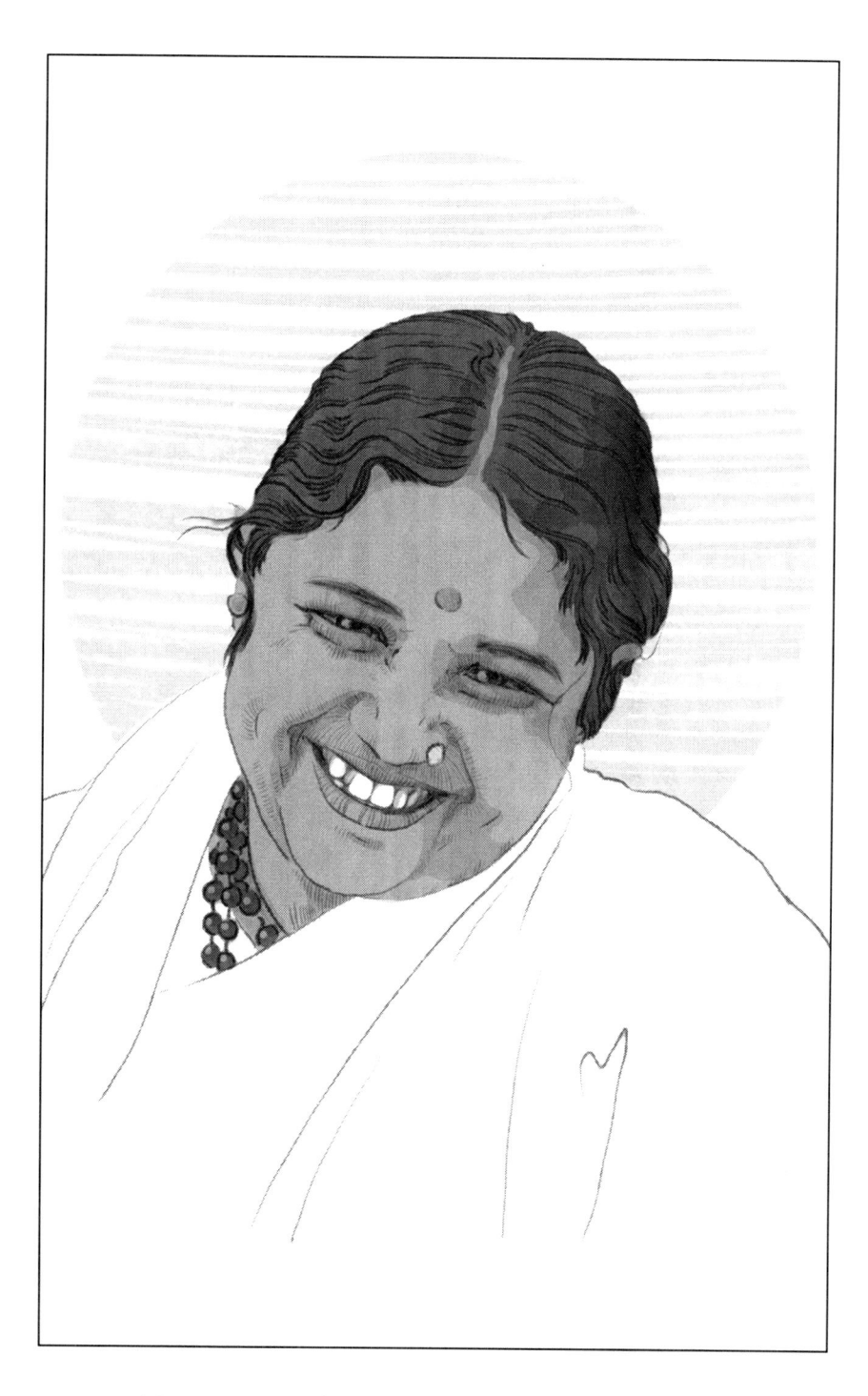

Mata Amritanandamayi – Amma. Drawing: Nanna Ernst

My first impression of Amma's ashram was lovely and peaceful. I had experienced many things on my way there and I really needed to rest. Although the communal singing was well under way when I arrived, a staff member still took the time to welcome me and show me around. She was kind and helpful and gave me a bucket and dipper so that I could take a bath straight away. After four hours in a crowded, hot, dusty and dirty local bus, the prospect of a bath was pure heaven.

Amma's main ashram consisted only of a large temple building and some low huts. A couple of hundred people at the most lived there ordinarily. The ashram is in Southern India on a small peninsula where it can get rather hot and humid. In the temple building there were sleeping quarters and a number of smaller apartments and rooms. Amma's helpers were pleasant and kind and the food was also adapted to western digestions.

When you live in an ashram, it is often appreciated if you carry out voluntary work on a daily basis f.ex. by giving a hand with some of the practical chores. On my first day at Amma's I was standing by a window wondering what I would like to do at this place. An Indian was watching me from a distance and eventually came and offered to do his work in cooperation with me. He told me that his home was in the US where as a professor he had studied and taught Indian spiritual philosophy. As he wanted to offer his work ability with the thing he most enjoyed doing, he offered to teach me these subjects. I was rather astounded at this offer, as it was almost the same offer I had previously been given by the German philosopher at Swamiji's ashram. I sent a loving thought to Swamiji, as he was the one who first asked me to learn some of these things. I gratefully accepted the offer, but only managed to have a couple of hours of lessons.

Unfortunately, I fell sick on the second day of my stay at Amma's ashram and my fever lasted the rest of my stay there. Every time the fever went down a little and I received a hug from Amma, my temperature immediately rose a few degrees. This showed me that a lot was happening energy wise during a hug of just a few seconds. But precisely because of the fever, the pains and the strong emotions which arose during this visit, I felt almost like a prisoner in her ashram. The fact that my reactions were so strong here may be an expression of the impact that Amma's state and powers had on me – a state of high intensity and vibration. Of course, it might also be a result of the preparatory work done via the visits with the other gurus. After seven days, I moved on although I was still running a high temperature. It was just time to leave.

There are also opportunities to meet Amma at other places outside India. Every year she travels to Europe, among other places, where she visits several towns in Germany and France. Stockholm has also been among her destinations a few times.

Papaji

Papaji was an elderly Northern Indian who at that time was 84 years old (born 1910). He is a student of the wellknown guru, Ramana Maharshi (1879-1946) who lived most of his life in his ashram by the mountain of Arunachala near Tiruvannamalai in Southern India. When he was quite young, Ramana had a revelation of self-realisation and became one with the divine. From this time on he transmitted peace and love from his whole being. It made people flock to him from far and near. Papaji is one of the few surviving students of Ramana. He also has spent many years showing people the path to their own inner divinity.

The story of how Papaji met his guru and later discovered the greatness of this man is very strange. I have written it here in my own words based on the description in source 27, pages 6-9.

When Papaji was eight years old, he had a spontaneous experience of being one with the divine. He was not able to describe the state or experience itself, but it made such a deep impression on him that afterwards he used all his energy on achieving it this state again.

Many Indians regard Krishna as the superior god. This was also the case for Papaji's mother. Therefore, she directed her son to use prayers and meditations addressed to Krishna as the means for helping him to achieve this state and become one with God again. Papaji practised night and day. The desired result failed to appear, but he carried on regardless. He even chose to give up his promising career with the military in order to concentrate on this burning desire. He asked all the so-called wise men whether they themselves or people they knew could show him Krishna, but nobody could help him. One day there was a knock at the door and a travelling god-seeking man – a sadhu – asked for food and drink. It is the custom in India to feed these people who have renounced all material things in their search for God. Papaji offered food to the stranger and seized the opportunity to ask whether he knew anyone who could show him God. Surprisingly enough, the guest replied that he knew a certain Ramana who lived about 3,000 km further south. This Master, Ramana, would be able to show him the way to his divine goal.

Papaji immediately packed his suitcase and set out. After a long and tiring journey he arrived weary and exhausted at Ramana's ashram. Papaji's first meeting with Ramana was not a positive experience. For instead of meeting God, he met his own anger. For Ramana turned out to be identical with the stranger who had knocked on Papaji's door in Northern India. Ramana did not answer his questions as to why he had deceived him and lured him into making this long journey. So Papaji packed his things again ready to go home. One of the other residents at the ashram came to him and asked why he was leaving again so soon. When he heard the answer, he told Papaji that Ramana had not left his town for more than

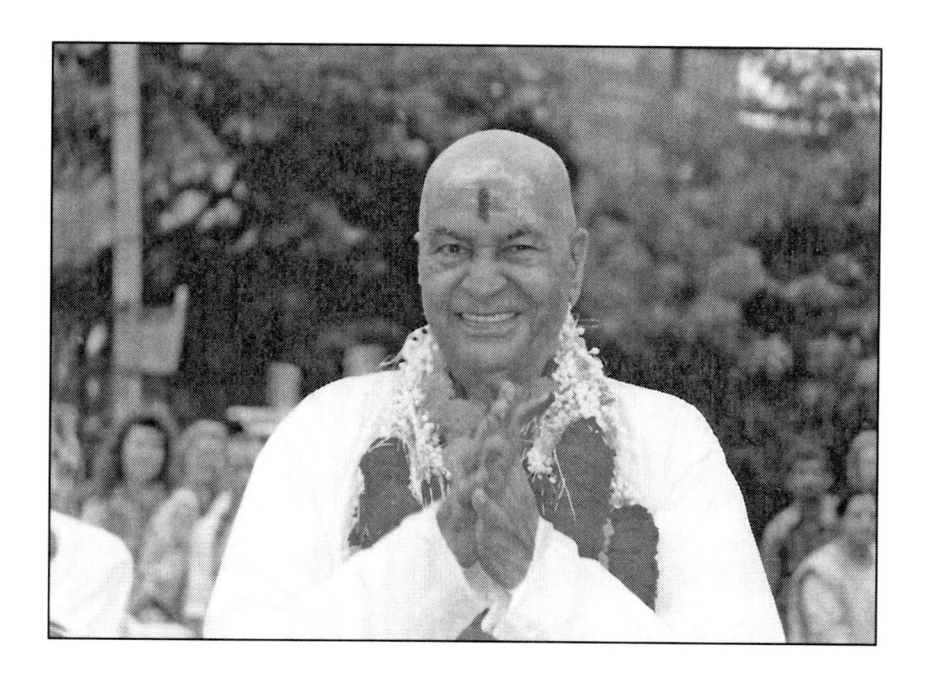

Poonjaji on his way from his home to the satsang room on his birthday. Photo: Lisbeth Ejlertsen from the visit in 1992

40 years. This made Papaji cool down a little and he stayed for a week or so. But even though he had a wonderful experience during a conversation with Ramana, he did not appreciate the manner of this Master. Therefore, he left the ashram and camped out on the other side of the mountain. There he meditated on Krishna and had some fascinating experiences of fooling around and playing with this God. On his way home he again stopped by at Ramana's ashram to brag about having met Krishna in his visions. Ramana's answer was:

"What is the use of a god who comes and goes again? If he really *is* God, he must stay with you *always*".

However, at this point Papaji was not prepared to hear and understand these words. He returned home and resumed his spiritual practice with meditation and reciting mantras. But after another few years of practice without achieving the desired result, it was no longer Krishna that he saw in his visions. It was the god Rama and one day also the guru

Ramana Maharshi. Then Papaji gave up his exercises and felt empty and disheartened. In his desperation he went to see Ramana again.

This time the meeting changed everything for Papaji. Ramana told him that his exercises had brought him here and had thus fulfilled their purpose. At this stage he no longer needed them and that was why he could not carry them out any more. It was not he who gave them up, but the exercises that left him. In this situation Papaji was now prepared to listen to and follow Ramana's advice. The guru looked at him intensely, and this look led Papaji to the insight or the place with which he had been in contact when he was eight years old. He had achieved his goal. This time it was not a short experience, but a permanent state of being which could not be described with words. And in this realisation, Papaji understood what Ramana had pointed out previously. That he should not link God with a particular image, such as Krishna, because all forms are transitory. Instead he should take an interest in the longing within himself from where he so passionately desired to meet God by asking and absorbing himself in the question: "*Who am I?*" Papaji came into contact with his own divinity, because in this way he directed his focus from the outer world towards the source within himself. Today, Papaji uses this same question, among other things, to support his followers in turning their focus toward their own Self.

Ramana Maharshi is the same guru to whom the English philosopher and mystic, Paul Brunton, returns again and again in his book "*A Search in Secret India*".

Unlike the other gurus, Papaji did not live in an ashram. Instead he offered his help by giving *satsang* a couple of hours each weekday in a house close to his home which was called "Satsangbhavan". The word "sat" means "existence" or "true", and the word "sang" means "meeting" or "gathering together". So "satsang" can be translated as "gathering together in truth". This refers to the fact that on these occasions the focus is directed on *truth* – that which always *is*.

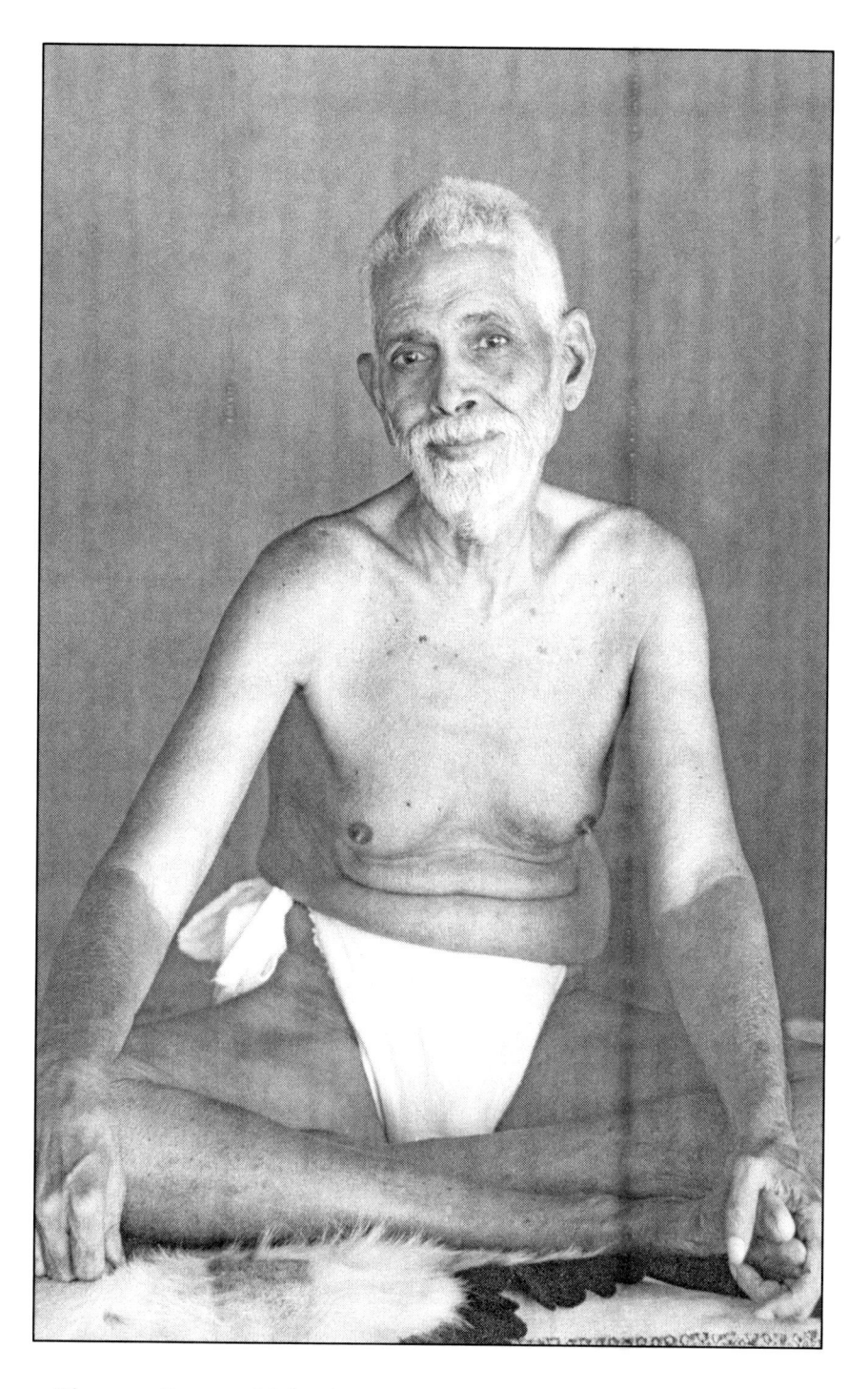

Bhagavan Ramana Maharshi, Poonjaji's guru. See source information VIII

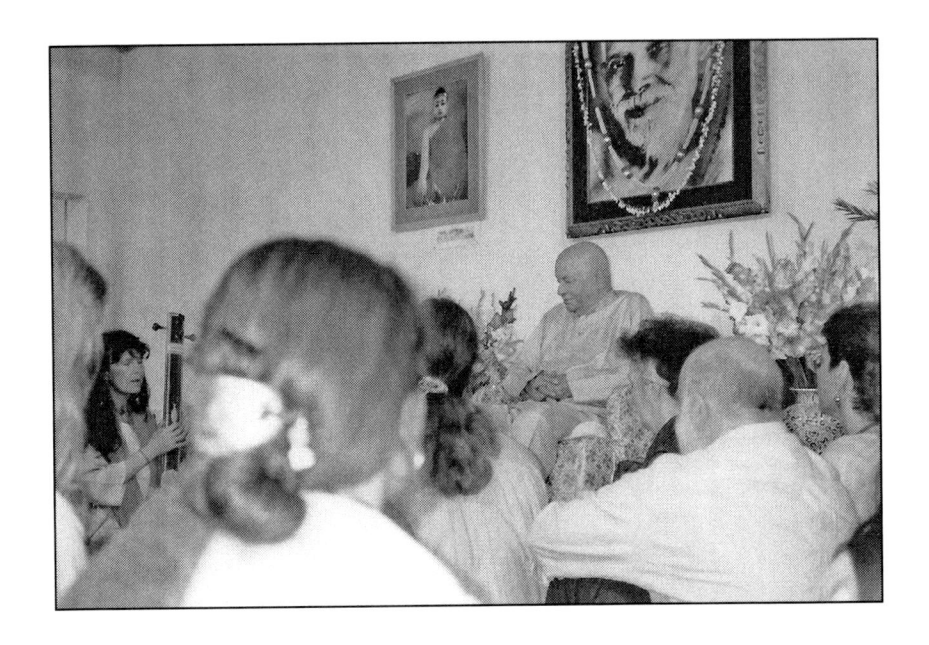

A satsang with Poonjaji is often concluded by someone performing with music or the like. Photo: Lisbeth Ejlertsen from the visit in 1992

At these satsangs Papaji placed himself at the disposal of the people in order to help them to recognise who they really are. Each person has to recognise the divine within him or herself, but Papaji did what he could to point them in the right direction. He did this by means of logical explanations without using ceremonies, mantras or songs. He guided people to seek liberation within themselves instead of remaining slaves of their thoughts, senses and feelings. As he pointed out, the idea is instead to see who we are behind all these disturbing elements. Papaji often compared the mind to a film screen. One moment it can be a horror film showing and the next a film about love. But when the film is over, the screen is still the same – untouched and unaffected by the dramas which were played out on it. In the same way the inner being is untouched by our thoughts, senses and feelings when and if we do not get involved with them. Therefore, he asks his students to shift their focus and attention away from the "films" in the physical world which we ourselves create or participate in. Instead we should direct this registration ability inwards to the place from which all experiences arise.

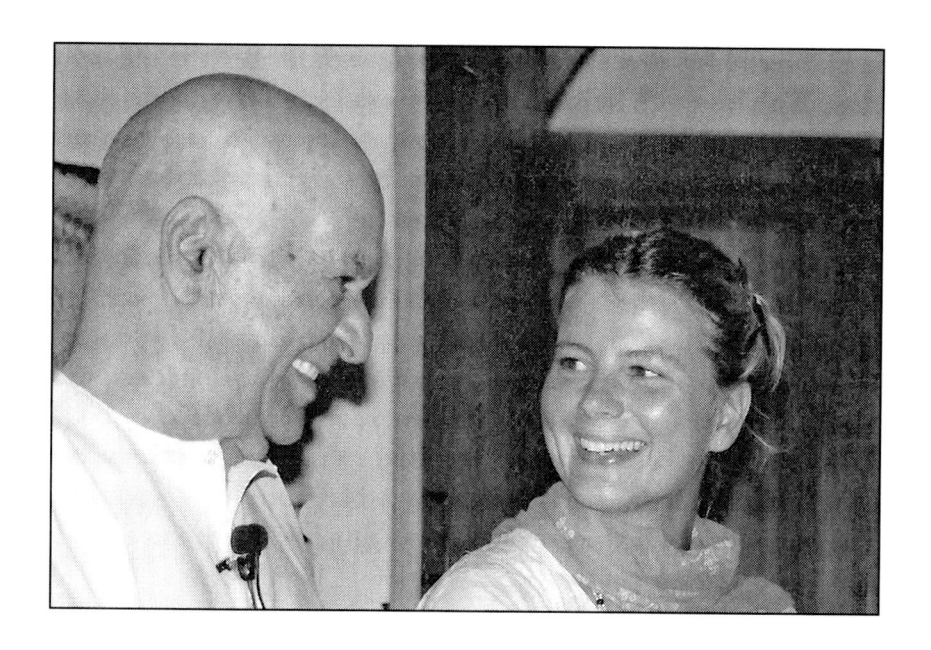

Poonjaji has just answered my questions and I was invited up to his side.
Photo: Unknown person who was present – from the visit in 1992

In other words Papaji encourages us to direct our gaze away from the "films" in the physical world and towards our inner "film screen" instead.

When Papaji was guiding his students by answering their questions, he was very clear-sighted, straightforward and direct. He understood how to see where people had got stuck and gave them a push in the right direction. Sometimes these pushes felt rather harsh, but even when he was scolding, he did it with love. It seemed that sometimes it was necessary to be harsh in order for people to understand the games they were playing with themselves. It *is* difficult not to think, because all our lives we have been brought up to understand that our mind is the most important thing. Therefore, provocation is necessary in some cases in order for people to take the first step and try something different. But in most cases, Papaji's manner was kind and caring.

During my first visit to Papaji in 1992 I had the opportunity – by asking him a question-to come and sit by his side. While he was answering my question with words, a lot was happening on a different level. I could feel that Papaji was guiding with his heart at the same time. With his words he made my brain wander in a certain direction. At the same time I sensed quite clearly an intense vibration in my heart. The effect of these two influences brought me for a short while into a space I will characterise as a state of *nothingness* outside time and place. I experienced my inner being as a greyish unlimited space of nothingness. At the same time as I was experiencing this inwardly, I was talking to Papaji. It was as if each word I was about to say loomed up in this space from nothing and as soon as I had seen and said this word, it dissolved again into nothingness and a new word loomed up. When I was not focussing on the words, the space was just empty, but even so filled with this greyish something which both was and was not. The experience lasted perhaps a couple of minutes. I began to wonder and Papaji pointed out that there was now "a big thought in front of me". He was right, for my wonder at this new inner state made me come out of it and I could not just go back to the same experience. This is the first and only time I have experienced the space of nothingness in this way. But it has left me with the realisation of the great difference between the inner state when it is just quiet and when the thoughts are receiving attention.

About 200 people, most of them foreigners, participated in a satsang with Papaji. Almost all countries and continents were represented: USA, Japan, Europe, Canada, Russia, Australia, New Zealand etc. Perhaps it is the very rational and logical mindset of this teacher that appeals so strongly to us foreigners. We often tend to choose that which seems logical rather than ceremonies as it is difficult for us to relate to them with our cultural background.

As mentioned, I had visited India before just to meet Papaji. I had met one of his students in Denmark and become so enthusiastic about his teaching that I wanted to experience the teacher for myself. Since then I have benefitted from using the tools he gave me and I only have positive things to say about Papaji and his teaching. Nevertheless, I felt that it was now time that I should work in new ways with spiritual energies and ideas – and from that grew the desire to meet the other gurus as well on this my second trip to India.

The addresses of the gurus

Below are the addresses and contact numbers for the four gurus' ashrams in India. They are all marked on the map of India in the first part of the book.

[2017: The following contact information has been updated in 2017. See also newer status for these gurus in chapter: "Postscript 2001 – 7 years after the trip" under "Newest facts about the gurus I visited in 1994".]

Swamiji's main ashram is about 100 km south-west of Bangalore in the middle of the southern tip of India. The address is:

Avadhoota Datta Peetha
Sri Ganapati Sachchidananda Ashram
Nanjangud Road
Datta Nagar
Mysore 570 025
INDIA
Tel.: +91-(0)821-2486 486
Internet address: http://www.dattapeetham.org

[NB! Sai Baba left this world on April 24th 2011. There are still activities going on in the Sai Baba organisation and in the main ashram at the address below.]

Sai Baba's main ashram is in the southern half of the country about 120 km north of the town of Bangalore. The address is:

Bhagawan Sri Sathya Sai Baba Ashram
Prasanthi Nilayam
Puttaparthi – 515134
Andra Pradesh
INDIA
Tel: +91-(0)8555-287390
Internet address: http://www.srisathyasai.org.in

Amma's main ashram is on a peninsula on the western side of the southern tip of India. The address is:

Mata Amritanandamayi Math
Amritapuri P.O.
690 546 Kollam
INDIA
Tel.: +91-476-289-7578
Tel.: +91-476-289-6399
Internet address to this ashram: http://www.amritapuri.org

American internet address: http://www.amma.org
Centers around the world: http://www.amma-europe.org/centres.html

[NB! Papaji left this world in the autumn of 1997. There are still activities going on at the addresses below.]

Papaji's home is situated in the north of India. The address is:

Papaji's House
20/144A
Indira Nagar
Lucknow
Uttar Pradesh-226016
INDIA
Tel.: +91-522-2348525
Tel.: +91-522-2348525

The address of the house where he gave satsang is:

Papaji Satsang Bhavan
A-306 Indira Nagar
Lucknow
Uttar Pradesh – 226016
INDIA
Internet address: http://www.satsangbhavan.net

BACK IN DENMARK

A completely different world ...

Now that I am back in Denmark again in this completely different world, my experiences in India can seem just like being in a dream. Because these two continents are so different, the reality of the one seems like a dream when I am in the other. But nevertheless, the reality of the journey is quite plain: The experiences are imprinted on my mind and in my soul. In general I will say that all four gurus showed me different aspects of divine wisdom and love. So my curiosity was satisfied after experiencing several gurus and thus fulfilling one of the goals of my journey. In particular, the charisma and nature of Swamiji are deeply imprinted in my heart. Not because I experienced him as a god, but because some of his charisma helped me to open my heart to more love. Being pervaded with love just gives one the desire and need to have even more. I have become addicted.

I thought that my journey was going to be a holiday in part, but it ended up being a pure study trip. I was gripped by the wisdom to be found in India and became quite a diligent student who simply could not get enough. It was as if I was constantly being led to the right places at the right times. I had not made sure that the gurus would be in their ashrams when I dropped by. Nevertheless, I succeeded in spending time with all four of them. I also received all kinds of help and support from people I knew as well as from strangers, so the journey was easy for me.

My aim to see a guru materialise objects out of thin air in front of my very eyes was not fulfilled. But it did not matter, because it was their message about seeking our inner divinity that was the most important thing.

The other goal of having my life story mapped out by a palm leaf astrologer was absolutely fulfilled. With these expectations met in full measure, one might think that I would be satisfied, and in fact I am. However, my curiosity and desire for new experiences has not been satisfied – on the contrary. I still feel drawn to this country which is so ugly and so beautiful at the same time. The inspiration I find in India is like a menu consisting of several dishes. None of them is expendable, because together they form a whole. Every time I finish a perfect meal, like now, I discover that I am still hungry. The physical disorders I had to suffer due to the dust and pollution cannot keep me from going back to this land of spiritual milk and honey.

When the first idea of a trip to India arose, it seemed to be financially quite impossible. Even so, perhaps because I was prepared to keep the dream in my heart, my situation changed completely and it became possible to make the trip. This also happened with all the goals I had set before starting out. They seemed to me to be quite ambitious before my departure. But in India I let the universe take control and the circumstances developed as I have related. My whole journey can be compared to this image: I chose to sow a spiritual seed of adventure even though it seemed unrealistic to me that it would be able to grow in the field I had at my disposal. But because I was open to the possibility and was vigilant when it needed care, the seed was miraculously able to take root and grow – and unfold like a fantastic fairy tale.

POSTSCRIPT 1997 – 3 YEARS AFTER THE TRIP

I meet a new Master and seek clarity

The journey I described here took place at the beginning of 1994 and I made the draft for this book immediately after. Before the manuscript was published, I came into contact with another Indian guru in 1995: *Chariji*. This meeting convinced me that he was to be my future spiritual mentor. As this book is my story of seeking wisdom and finding mentors, I find it relevant to round it off by mentioning him and the meditation system, *Sahaj Marg*, which he teaches.

[Today the word "Heartfulness" is used as the entrance portal to the meditation system Sahaj Marg. See more on this in the postscript "Postscript 2017 – 23 years after the trip".]

My meeting with Chariji took place in 1995 at a summer seminar in Jutland. In India they say that when you yourself are ready, your guru will come to you. This for me is a wonderful example of the humour of the universe, because I travelled almost to the ends of the earth to seek what I finally found here in Denmark. There were about 2,000 participants at the seminary that summer, so it might be a bit much to claim that the guru came to *me* there – but all the same …

In this postscript the emphasis is also on creating clarity regarding spiritual questions to which I myself have sought answers. My meeting with the gurus and the Indian spiritual philosophy in 1994 gave me a framework on which to build my understanding. But there were still many specific questions which were important for me to have clarified. Some of these were:

- Is it necessary to have a Master in order to develop spiritually?
- Why is it important to have just one Master if you wish to attain the spiritual goal?
- How can you find your Master and how do you choose the "right one" among the many?
- Is it necessary to meditate in order to develop spiritually?
- What is the difference between "the mind" and "the Soul" in us human beings?
- How does a Master describe the divine state?
- What is the quickest way for me to attain the spiritual goal?
- Why is the meditation system Sahaj Marg so special?

Satisfactory answers to such questions can only be given by Masters who can speak from their own experiences. The answers which I have found and included in this postscript are excerpts from writings and speeches by the two Masters, Chariji and Babuji. As mentioned, Chariji is the mentor I have chosen and Babuji was Chariji's predecessor and Master.

Initially, I still prefer to learn through experience. Just as on my journey to India, I spontaneously follow the path which my heart points to. Not until then do I find the explanations which the intellect needs in order to accept what happens.

After my meeting with Chariji it became even more urgent for me to have the above questions clarified. So I started reading the literature concerning the meditation system Sahaj Marg and the Masters. Before sharing the experiences from my meeting with Chariji at the seminar in 1995, I will pass on the answers to these questions – but not in the order listed. For a description of certain words and concepts must be available before they can be part of the answer to other questions. It has been my priority that the answers and the description of Chariji and of the meditation system, Sahaj Marg, should come in a natural and easily comprehensible sequence.

Only some of the source material from the two Masters is available in Danish; the rest is in English. Therefore, I have translated most of the following extracts myself. I make certain reservations here for any errors which might occur in translation.

The Master Chariji

Chariji's full name is Shri Parthasarathi Rajagopalachari. He is normally called *Chari, Chariji* or *Master,* Master being the English version of the word "guru". The name by which this Master goes is a short version of his surname, as "chari" consists of the last five letters of his surname since the whole name is rather difficult to pronounce. In India, the ending "ji" is often added to a person's name when wishing to express respect for the person in question. Thus the name Chariji.

In 1995 Chariji was a 68 year old, (born 1927), extremely humorous and talented gentleman. In his earlier working life he had been a much-travelled and successful business man – now he was a much-travelled and successful Master. Chariji was 36 years old when he encountered the Sahaj Marg meditation system, and later that same year his Master Babuji. On the outer level Chariji continued for many years carrying out his duties to his job and his family. At the same time he worked on the inner levels through the daily practice and contact with the Master. This transformed his personality and inner capacity to such an extent that Babuji appointed him as his successor. In April 1983, Babuji left his physical body (1899-1983); Chariji was 55 years old at the time. Since then Chariji has been the Master for this meditation practice and he has devoted the rest of his life to supporting people in their spiritual development.

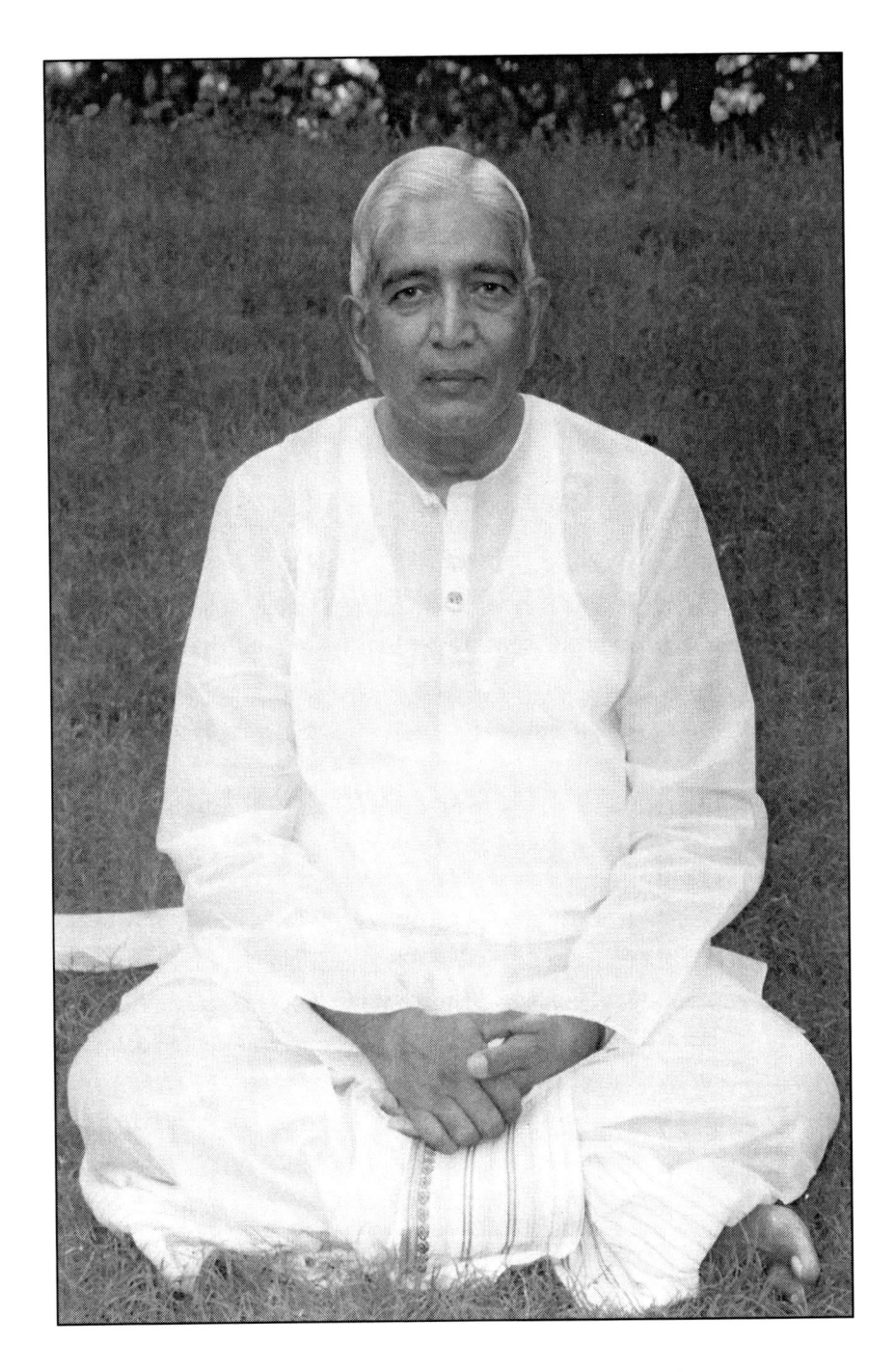

P. Rajagopalachari – Chariji. See source IX

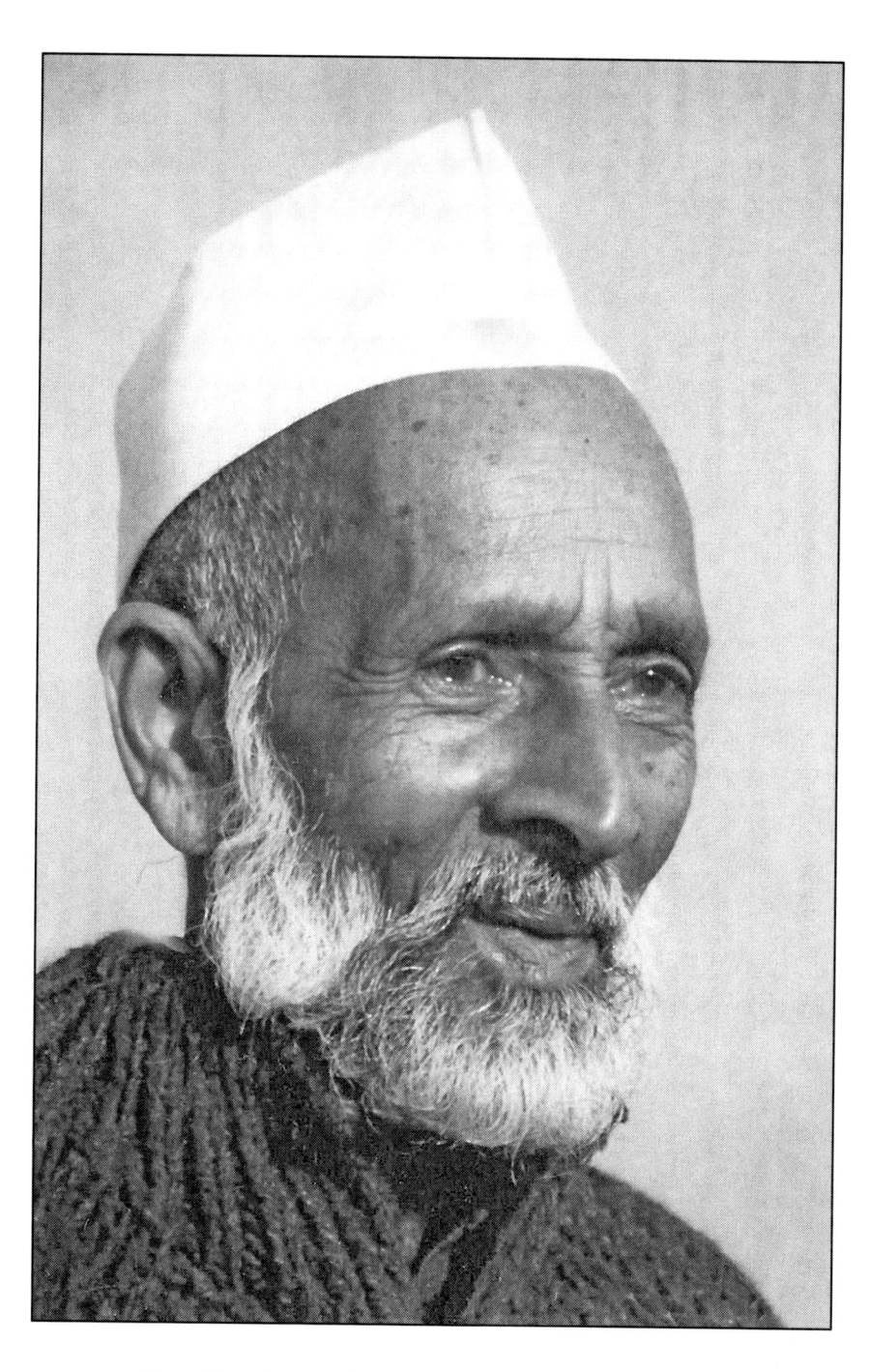

Ram Chandra – Babuji – Chariji's Master. See source IX

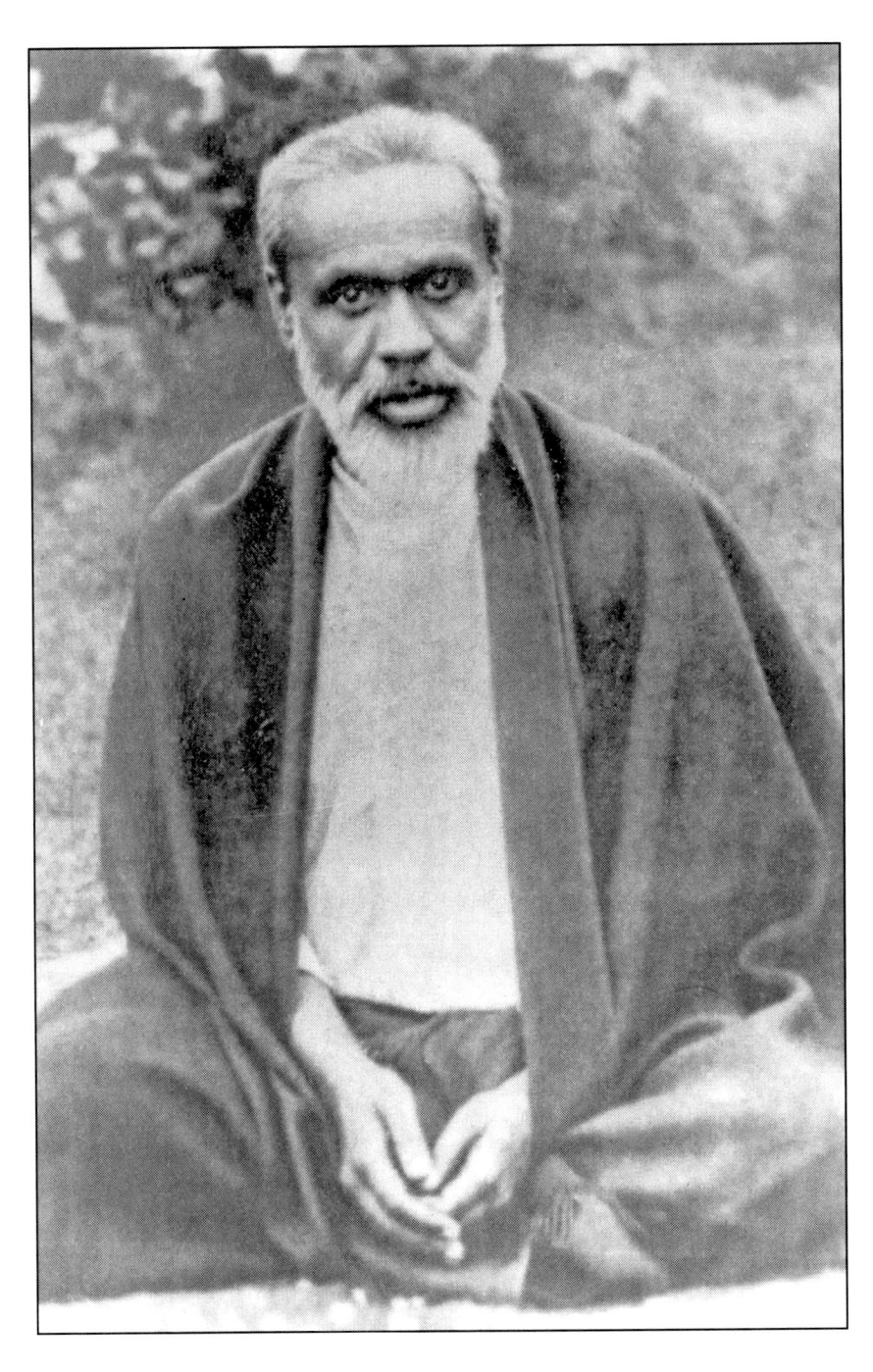

Ram Chandra – Lalaji – Babuji's Master and the first Master in this lineage. See source IX

Babuji also had a Master, ordinarily called *Lalaji,* (1873-1931). Lalaji was the actual founder of this system of meditation. "Lalaji" and "Babuji" are also just "nicknames" for these two gurus. In this case their nicknames were very useful, because both their Indian first and surnames were the same – both were called Ram Chandra and both came from Northern India. Lalaji came from Fatehgarh and Babuji from Shahjahanpur. Thus Chariji is the third Master in this system. He lives in the southern part of India in Chennai, a large city previously called Madras. The main centre for this system is today placed in a town near to Chennai called Manapakkam.

Chariji recommends his students to follow a daily practice and this is where he differs significantly from the other four gurus I visited in India. In order to understand this approach to spiritual development and Chariji's work as a Master, it is necessary to know a little about both the practical and the philosophical aspect of Sahaj Marg which is outlined below.

As an introduction I will tell about my own introduction to this system of meditation. Just as it happened to Chariji, I also was introduced to the mediation system before I met the Master. This is how it happened:

My introduction to Sahaj Marg

I encountered Sahaj Marg about a year after my return from India. At that time I had had a great desire for about 6 months to meditate by a different method than the ones I already knew. After my return from India I had put my whole heart and a great deal of will into meditating with a long mantra which was in daily use with the guru Swamiji. After about 3 months of persevering practice, I had finally learnt the mantra by heart. Even so I found that this mantra was very strenuous to recite and I did not feel any noticeable effect. One day I came across the Gayatri mantra. It is much shorter and was a lot easier to use, so in my daily practice I exchanged the long mantra for the Gayatri mantra.

After a few months of practising this mantra I still felt no immediate results from my efforts. Although the Gayatri mantra was somewhat easier to use, I was still a little bored during the daily recitation. Before my trip I had just been meditating by myself for many years, but neither did this approach appeal to me any more. I needed new inspiration which first and foremost would give perceptible results ...!

I had not shared my thoughts on finding a new meditation practice with anyone. One day I met one of my friends who told me surprisingly that she had just been introduced to a method of meditation. The funny thing about this was that she had asked me several times to teach her to meditate. Although I had given her a positive answer each time, nothing ever came of it. Now instead, she was the one who came to teach me about this form of meditation, Sahaj Marg, to which she had been introduced. Her enthusiasm aroused my curiosity. Together we watched a video about Chariji and the system. The same evening I telephoned the person who had introduced the system to my friend. Thus the path was opened for me to try it as well. My wish to meditate sprang from a deep desire to find the peace and calm within myself. It was not a result of theoretical explanations about the advantages of meditation. So I went to this introduction with a curious mind and with my senses open.

Transmission – the unique aspect of Sahaj Marg

What is unique about Sahaj Marg is the fact that the students' own meditation practice is combined with transmission from the Master. The transmission is given in the course of a *sitting* during which one or more students sit opposite the guru while the latter administers the divine state into the hearts of those present. If there is only one student in front of Chariji, the sitting is called an *individual sitting*. If there is more than one student receiving transmission, it is called a *group sitting*.

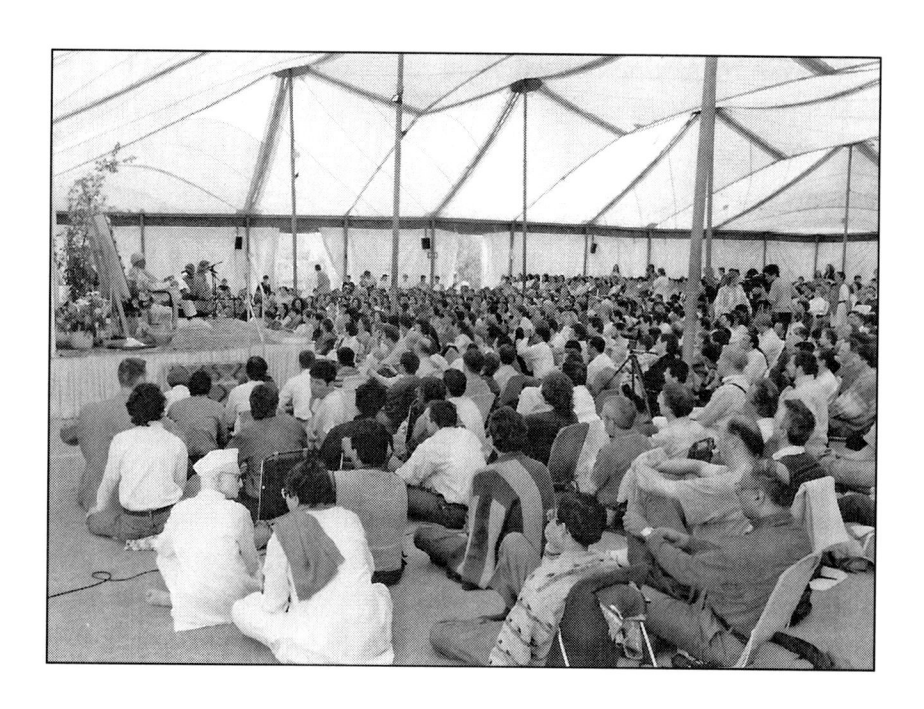

Just after a large group sitting with Chariji. See source X

To be able to transmit the divine essence is a special technique called pranahuti in the Raja Yoga system. That is why transmission is also called "pranahuti" or "yogic transmission". Only a few yogis of high calibre have had the capacity to be able to transmit, and this technique had long been forgotten in India until it was rediscovered by Lalaji – the first Master of this Sahaj Marg system.

During a transmission, the divine state – which is very subtle – is created in the students' hearts and there this fine and light quality is established. This subtle and "energy-less" energy will awaken and nourish the seed of our own divinity which is to be found precisely there. The aim for the Master is to support each person in developing his or her own contact with the divine essence – so that the seed in each student's heart will grow into a strong and healthy plant. In this way, reception of the transmission becomes an aid to the spiritual development of the aspirant. At the same time this illustrates that the task of the Master is to help the student follow the path on his own – not by placing himself as an intermediary, but by "pushing" the student forwards via the transmission. With this help the Master promises that it is possible to achieve God-realisation in the course of just one life.

When Chariji is not physically present himself, the transmission flows through one of his helpers who sits in his place in front of the recipients. The helpers are called *preceptors*. Their task is to act as channels for the Master's transmissions. In this situation they can be regarded as his extended arm or rather perhaps his extended heart, because it is always Chariji himself who gives the sitting through their hearts. When the Master prepares a preceptor, he cleanses the heart of that person so that it becomes a pure channel. After that a preceptor can easily give a transmission to another student who might even be spiritually more developed. For the transmission is unaffected by the preceptor's own spiritual capacity – it just flows from the Master through this preceptor to the recipient. Therefore, the preceptors do not form an extra hierarchy in the organisation, but are a natural part of the student group. At the time of writing there are more than 30 preceptors in Denmark.

Transmission can also be given at a distance. This means that a preceptor can be anywhere in the world and give a transmission to a person who might be in their own home, for example. This is a result of the Master's capacity which in some inexplicable way reaches outside time and place.

Thus the Sahaj Marg system depends on the techniques transmission and meditation. Here a student is called an "abhyasi". This word from Sanskrit means quite simply "one who practises".

Lalaji, who rediscovered the transmission, had such a great spiritual capacity that he attained divine realisation in just seven months – without the help of any Master. His successor, Babuji, combined Lalaji's knowledge and the ability to transmit. Among other things, Babuji defined the daily practice which the students – *abhyasis* – also carry out today. In 1945, Babuji founded the association Shri Ram Chandra

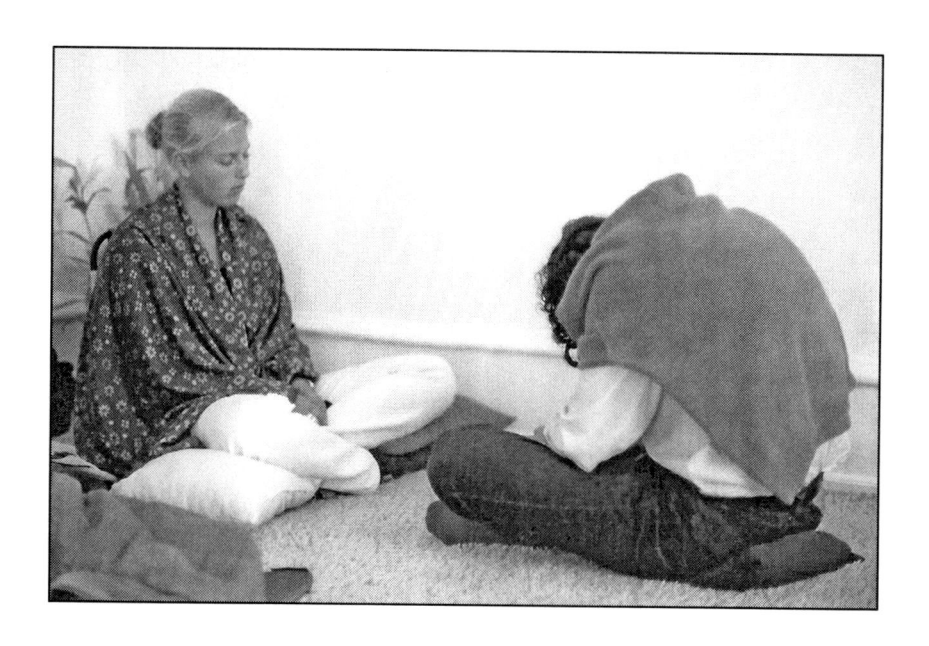

*An individual sitting where the receiver is deeply
absorbed in meditation. See source X*

Mission which he named after his Master. This association, which in Denmark is known by the abbreviation SRCM, has since formed the outer framework for this spiritual work.

In order to spread the knowledge of Sahaj Marg, Babuji travelled around in and outside India. On his first journey abroad in 1972, which went to both Europe and the US, Denmark was one of his destinations. He was particularly fond of the Danish abhyasis who also visited him in India. Chariji, who as mentioned is the third Master of Sahaj Marg, also travels round the world to develop spiritual potential everywhere. He also loves coming to Denmark. Almost every summer he spends a short week in the Jutland town of Vrads about 17 km south west of Silkeborg. This is where one of the two ashrams to be found in Europe lies. The other is in the French town of Augerans in the mid-eastern part of the country. The combined great efforts of the three Masters to make the system accessible to everyone have borne fruit. Today there are Sahaj Marg centres on all the continents in the world.

The Sahaj Marg meditation system in practice

"Sahaj Marg" means "the natural way" or "the simple way". Naturalness and simplicity are exactly the characteristics of this system which can be combined with an ordinary life. The daily practice consists of a meditation in the morning, an inner cleaning in the evening and a prayer at bedtime. There is actually an emphasis on living a normal family life and active participation in the community, because, among other things, being with others constitutes the best place for learning spiritual development. The individual elements in Sahaj Marg, which will all be described in more detail below, can be summarised as follows:

The abhyasis' own practice:

- daily meditation in the morning, 1 hour
- daily cleaning in the evening, ½ hour
- daily prayer before bedtime, 10 min.
- practice during the day in being in the state of *Constant Remembrance*

Other activities:

- individual sittings; receiving an individual sitting of about ½ hour about every 2 weeks
- group sittings; participation in a group sitting of about 1 hour about once a week
- being with the Master – preferably once a year, for example at a seminar

The fact that this system can be practised by everyone who is interested is described by Chariji as follows:

"Prospective entrants to this system invariably ask one question, "What are the qualifications required to be a member of this system?" Master's

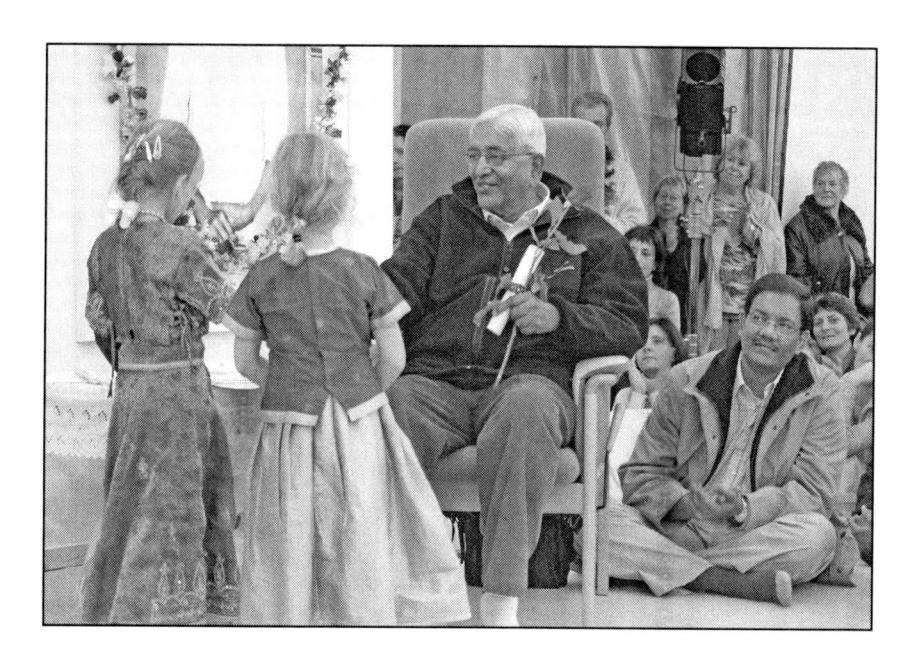

During a visit to Denmark Chariji was given a rose and song lyrics by the youngest children. The music event with a children's choir took place after a group sitting. Photo: Lisbeth Ejlertsen

[Babujis] only answer to this question is, "Your willingness is the only qualification needed."" (see source 37 p. 33)

The underlying philosophy of Sahaj Marg

The aim of Sahaj Marg is to support the individual in transforming his or her inner state towards the divine state which is infinitely fine and subtle. Babuji explains the aim as follows:

"What we must strive for in order to secure absolute freedom from bondage is to become the lightest and the finest, closely corresponding with the

godly attributes and securing complete similarity with Him. The nectar of real life is for him and him alone who brings himself up to the standard required for the purpose." (see source 31 p. 19)

The aim can be achieved by a combination of the abhyasis' own efforts and the support of the Master. Babuji describes this with the following encouragement:

"I may assure you very sincerely that realization is not at all a difficult thing, if you earnestly divert your attention to it. Iron will to achieve the goal together with proper means and guidance is the only thing required for the complete success." (see source 31 p. 65)

Sahaj Marg's connection with Raja Yoga

As mentioned, it was the Masters Lalaji and Babuji who developed the systemised use of transmission and cleaning which is used in Sahaj Marg. These are quite special tools which, as far as I know, are only used in this system. But the underlying philosophy of the meditation – sitting with eyes closed and allowing the attention to rest on one place – has roots back in the time of the Vedas and parallels to Raja Yoga. As previously mentioned, Patañjali called the seventh step in his yoga system Raja Yoga – the part which shows how to process and manage the mind through meditation. The word "raja" means "kingly" or "noble", and Babuji writes as follows on the meaning of this name:

"The kingly thing in us is thought which ultimately develops, steering us to our goal." (see source 30 p. 122)

The basis for Raja Yoga is that the human power of thought is related to the vibration with which this world was created. Because the power of thought is creative in essence, it can – by the means of meditation – be used to transform the mind. This is why Sahaj Marg starts from exactly this part of the yoga system. Babuji and Chariji, respectiviely explain as follows:,

"Under the Sahaj Marg system of training we start from Dhyana, the seventh step of yoga fixing our mind on the point in order to practice meditation. The previous steps are not taken up separately, but they automatically come into practice as we proceed on with meditation. Thus, much of our time and labour is saved by this means." (see source 31 p. 98)

"No preparation whatsoever is needed for a person to begin meditation because as Master [Babuji] *has emphasized again and again, meditation is an instrument for the purification of the mind and its preparation for communion with the Ultimate. That is, meditation is a means to an end and not an end in itself. This being so, anybody who is willing to try it or practice it is qualified by that very willingness, and needs no further preparation or qualification."* (see source 43 p. 165)

Briefly about the cleaning in Sahaj Marg

The word "cleaning" is used about the purifying process which an abhyasi carries out in the evening when the work of the day is finished. The purpose of the *cleaning* is to cleanse the mind of impressions. Cleaning can roughly be compared to a shower – only it is the mind and the heart that are cleaned by this process. Cleaning is done as follows: You sit in a comfortable position, close your eyes and imagine that all the impressions of the day – all impurities and complexities – disappear out of your back like smoke or steam. You imagine that the smoke and steam can leave the body via the whole of the back from the top of the head to the end of the tailbone. When the impurities leave body and mind in this way, a vacuum is created inside the whole body. Now you imagine that this vacuum has become filled with the subtlest of light with the finest vibration – the so-called divine light. You can either let it stream from the innermost core of your heart or, if you imagine that the Master is sitting in front of you during the cleaning, this subtlest of light can come from His heart. When the cleaning is finished, the whole body if filled with light and lightness.

As human beings we are exposed to many influences every day. This takes places from the inside via our own thoughts and feelings and from the outside by being with other people. These influences form patterns and impressions on our mind, some of which may border on the traumatic. In Sanskrit, these impressions on the mind are called *samskaras*. The purpose of cleaning all the samskaras away is to make the mind completely neutral so that our doings can be free and not controlled by earlier impressions. Only through a pure mind can the light shine clearly in us and through us.

During our daily cleaning which takes 20-30 minutes it is mainly only the impressions from the same day which are removed. We must have help to rid ourselves of the deep impressions which may originate both from this life and previous lives. This help is given during a sitting when the preceptor spends time cleaning the abhyasi. The vibration during a transmission is so intense and has such a subtle quality, that it can gradually resolve everything which impedes the spiritual development of the abhyasi.

My own experience with the cleaning method is that even when I am completely tired out and exhausted before this cleaning, I always feel very much refreshed afterwards. Again this can be compared to the freshness which the body feels externally after a shower. Therefore I am always happy to carry out the cleaning at the end of the day's work. Even if I only have a short time available of perhaps 5-10 minutes, the cleaning has a great effect. Sometimes, if for example something has had a very emotional impact on me at some point during the day, I sometimes choose to carry out a short cleaning process in the situation itself. This brings my mind into balance again – or at least part of the way there.

Definition of "the Self" and "the mind"

The Self is just another word for the soul which is the eternal and unchanging element in us all. It is present, regardless of whether we are present here on earth in a physical body, or whether we exist on another level. About the soul, Babuji says:

"The existence of soul can be traced out as far back as to the time of creation when the soul existed in its naked form as a separate entity." (see source 31 p. 21)

The mind can be approximately defined as the inner space where thoughts and feelings unfold. It is in the mind that ideas arise and it is here that we create our opinions and make rules about this and that. The mind forms not only the framework for what is happening in the now – it also affects our behaviour in the now through the previous personal experiences which lie hidden in our minds. In this way our past impacts to a great extent on our present thoughts and reactions and thus on our lives. Thus the mind plays a significant part in creating the personality. In some cases the mind is so overburdened that it pathologically distorts the received impressions. Ordinarily, we call people in this situation mentally ill – sick in their minds.

The mind always wants to attract our attention – and be the only centre in our personal universe. It keeps on creating activity with thoughts, feelings, considerations etc. so it can keep our attention in this way. In fact the untamed mind keeps us bound to our heads and thus away from the heart and from meeting the soul there.

There is quietness when we allow the mind to rest. We only achieve quietness in the mind when we do not give our attention to thoughts, feelings bodily sensations or other distractions. People do not often experience this quietness, because our immediate tendency is to fill the mind with activity. Only in quietness can the Self unfold and show that it exists and is one with everything. When we are in contact with the Self, we are in contact with the divine state. Therefore, a calm and neutral mind is a necessary step on the way to exploring the Self and – ultimately – to freeing us from the illusions of this world and achieving realisation.

When, through training via meditation, we achieve control over the mind so it does not "catch" our attention, but is instead trained to work for us, then we can benefit from this mind which is also a unique tool which is necessary to arrive at realisation. The Master Chariji expresses it in this way:

"The mind is our enemy, but the mind is also the only instrument through which we can gain this victory and make sure that human birth makes use of this very valuable opportunity on earth to achieve the goal of human birth, which is to gain liberation from it." (See source 44 p.111)

The difference between what the mind and the Self are in humans is brilliantly illustrated by the following well-known image: It also shows the effect it has on the mind when thoughts are repeated again and again. The example is partly quoted from source 28 p. 11.

The mind is like a woodland lake. The Self is like the bottom of the lake. When the surface of the water is completely still, one can clearly see the bottom: one can have insight into the Self. The impact of thoughts can be compared to waves on the surface of the water. When they are there, the image of the bottom is distorted. *"The waves not only disturb the surface of the water, they also build up sand banks at the bottom of the lake by constant repetition. Such sand banks naturally become more permanent than the waves themselves. They can be compared to tendencies and latent states which exist in the subconscious and unconscious areas of the mind. In Sanskrit these banks are called samskaras. Samskaras are built up from the effects of repeated thought waves and they then create new thought waves again. In this way the process works in both directions. If you submit the mind to constantly angry thought waves, you will discover that they build up angry samskaras which then again act on your behalf to find an opportunity for a burst of anger in your daily life ... In fact it can be said that our character at a given moment in time is formed by the sum of our samskaras".*

In some of the Upanishads the Self, and how to obtain access to the Self, is expressed in a more poetic form. The following beautiful description originates from the Kaivalya Upinashad:

"Earth, water, fire, air, ether I have none. Knowing the true nature of the Supreme Self, the one who dwells in the cave of the heart, without impurities, without duality, the universal witness, free from (the distinction of) being and non being, one attains the being of the Supreme Self." (see source 21 verse 23)

Meditation in Sahaj Marg

The daily meditation of the abhyasis is carried out as follows: You sit in a relaxed position with your eyes closed. You start by assuming that your heart is already filled with divine light – you imagine that the aim for the meditation has already been successfully achieved. The designation "divine light" is used as a description of the subtlest vibration and state that exist. Such an assumption works on many levels where it clears the path for attaining the highest state in the heart. Divine light is not to be visualised, otherwise it would limit the goal to what is known and can be imagined beforehand – to that which exists in the physical world. Divine light is beyond the physical world.

After assuming the divine light, you just remain still and direct your awareness to the region of your heart where you stay watchful of what might unfold there. It is an exercise in being patient and trusting that the innermost core of your heart – the divine source there – will spontaneously attract your attention to itself. Therefore, you do not have to do anything, neither in thought or action. There is no concrete goal to be achieved! The goal itself is the "process" as a whole as well as the act of directing your attention inwards and experiencing what happens. In the words of an ancient proverb you become what you meditate on. Meditation is a period of time in which you focus on being close to your innermost being – the Self – which you just have to be open to discovering and experiencing.

In order to maintain this state of watchfulness, you need to let go of any tension. It is the nature of thoughts to always be streaming ahead. During meditation the art is to leave them in peace and not give them any attention. If you discover that you are in the middle of a train of thought, you just let it go and return again to being watchful in your heart. It is a very important ground rule in Sahaj Marg that the mind must not be strained in any way. Therefore thoughts must not be suppressed, but must gently be let go. Any strain will just create new traces in the mind which then also have to be cleaned away.

Some of Babuji's own instructions about meditation are as follows:

"The method of meditation on the heart is to think of Godly light within it. When you begin meditating in this way please think only that Godly light within is attracting you. Do not mind if extraneous ideas haunt you during meditation. Let them come but go on with your own work. Treat your thoughts and ideas as uninvited guests." (see source 29 p. 333)

The reason that the heart is chosen as the focal point in Sahaj Marg meditation is explained by Babuji as follows:

"The heart is the pumping station of the blood. It sends out blood, after purification, to different nerves and cells of the body. Now we have taken the heart as the centre of meditation. The blood that runs throughout our system is affected. The solidity due to our own thoughts and actions begins

to melt away. This is the first thing we begin to gain, from the very first day, by this method of meditation on the heart." ...

"Whenever the idea of heart comes to them they locate its position as that of the heart made of the things said above. This is one of the limitations in viewing the Heart Region in its broader sense. It is really a vast circle covering everything inner and outer ... The stages of human approach are lying hidden in it;" ...

"It is the main artery of God. We cannot reach Him unless we proceed through it." (see source 30 pp. 131 and 134)

That meditation is simultaneously an observing and a dynamic process is explained by Chariji as follows:

"... many people just go into meditation and start snoring and they are not aware of anything else. It is done in a mechanical way. And they enjoy the meditation rather than do the meditation. And Babuji used to say, "This is a mechanical thing and they have no progress at all." Because when we meditate, it has to be a dynamic process in which the goal is always in our view. That is, a movement towards the goal is involved." (see source 36 p. 50)

Chariji also stresses that the aim of meditation is to control the mind so that we are the ones using the mind as a tool for our development instead of allowing the mind to go its own way and thus misuse our time and energy:

"So meditation is a process, it is not an end in itself. I say this because I find often preceptors say, "Meditate and everything is solved." Nothing is solved by meditation. By meditation, we meditate. What do we achieve by meditation? Then if people ask, you see, by mastering the ability to think continuously of something, I gain a regulatory control over my own mind. I have now the possibility of applying that mind where I choose. It is able to reveal to me the truth of whatever I seek. So at its peak, meditation can

do nothing but serve as an instrument of revelation, because the mind is perfected, the mind is regulated, and the mind becomes one-pointed and now I can use it for everything except to know God. Because God, not being an object, cannot be the object of concentration." (see source 36 p. 50)

What is meditation actually?

In his scripture: The Yoga Sutra, Patañjali, the father of yoga gave his definition of the concept of meditation which he calls "Dhyana". The definition is quoted below from a direct translation from Sanskrit to English and is as close as possible to the source:

"In meditative absorption, the entire perceptual flow is aligned with that object." (see source 45 p. 39 item III.2)

It may be easier to understand it via Vyasa's comment in source 46:

"Meditation is the continuance, i.e., the unchanging flow, of the mental effort to understand the object of meditation, untouched by any other effort of the understanding." (see source 46 p.180)

Babuji, whose knowledge is based on his direct insight into nature which is the true source, describes meditation as follows:

"Under the Sahaj Marg system of training we start from "dhyan", the seventh step of Patañjali yoga, fixing our mind on one point in order to practice meditation." (see source 29 p. 331)

The art of fixing the mind on one thing and not allowing yourself to be distracted by thought requires training. Because when you sit down with your eyes closed to meditate, most people will quickly discover that their thoughts jump around all over the place in an often unpredictable and never-ending chain of thought. One thought replaces the next without any pause in between, and the tendency to dwell on them is strong. Particularly in the West, being able to think and theorise is associated with high status. Therefore, we have a strong tendency to fix our awareness on the thoughts. And as long as our flickering thoughts receive our attention, we prevent ourselves from exploring the Self.

By meditating daily you can practise not involving yourself in your thoughts and then they will slide away of their own accord. For in reality, nobody and nothing can steal our attention – at the end of the day we are the only ones who can decide where we will direct our focus. When our sights are fixed on the source of divine light in the innermost core of our hearts – instead of on the contents of our thoughts – pauses will gradually occur between the thoughts and the connection to them will become less. Through regular training you will soon discover that your thoughts become less disturbing and that your tranquillity increases. Finally, unnecessary thoughts will disappear completely; the surface of the water will remain untouched and the bottom of the lake will be visible; you will be at one with the divine state.

There are many different systems of meditation which each make use of their own meditation practice. Not all methods are in harmony with the original purpose of meditation. In Sahaj Marg it is essential not to make use of concentration or control during meditation. Such heavy-handed methods violate the mind and make it stiff and inflexible and thus not open. This applies to the rough methods where control is used to restrain the mind by using a mantra or an external object. Hard bicycle training can make the cyclist's calf muscles suited to bicycle racing, but at the same time they will become stiff and inflexible which will make them unsuitable for many other activities. Similarly, the mind must not become stiff and inflexible. For if you wish to become one with the divine, which is infinitely fine and subtle, the mind must be the same; it must be flexible in every respect. Restraining the mind by force is like throwing stones in the woodland lake. It creates recognisable patterns on the surface, but the patterns have nothing to do with the bottom – the Self. Observing these patterns is not the same as acknowledging the Self and thus experiencing reality. Babuji explains this as follows:

"The real solution of the problem lies, not in controlling the mind artificially by suppression, restraint or mortification, but in its gradual moulding which is to relieve it of its misdirected trends." ...

"Concentration is the automatic and natural result of meditation. Those who insist on concentration in place of meditation, and force their mind to it, generally meet with failure." ...

"If we concentrate on a solid thing we are sure to become ourselves inwardly solid." (see source 29 pp. 335 and 333 and source 31 p. 16)

Practising meditation is an aid to getting rid of habit-bound thoughts. When they disappear, the divinely inspired impulses have room to come forward and be useful. Achieving quietness of mind is not in itself the final goal. This is where the soul starts its journey towards God which is infinite, because God is infinite. Basically, the realisation process is indescribable, because it can only be experienced. When in spite of this we try to communicate purpose and path with a single image such as the woodland lake, some limitations and incorrectness are introduced. The woodland lake example can give the impression that all thinking has a negative impact. This is not the case as the energy of thought, as previously mentioned, can be compared to the creative energy. Thinking is the necessary tool of the will in order to achieve the goal. The tendency to want to be able to understand the context of things is strong, but any descriptive image must be let go again, because spiritual development is also about being open to not knowing what we do not know, that is to acknowledge the limitations of knowledge and instead release the brain and open up for the unknown in our hearts.

Why meditation is a necessary instrument

The parts of our being as a human with which we are in contact during meditation are the mind and the Self – the latter can roughly be called "the soul". It is the mind that can pave the way via the heart and open the gateway to the soul and to unification with the divine state. In order to achieve realisation one must first of all go through this gateway and meet the soul. It is the mind's willingness to co-operate which will be ripened and refined through spiritual development. Meditation is an aid to opening the gateway and crossing the bridge from the mind to the soul.

The whole purpose and usefulness of meditation is explained very simply by Babuji as follows:

"The answer is quite plain and simple, that by meditation we gather ourselves at one point so that our indiviual mind may leave its habit of wandering about, which it has formed. By this practice we set our individual mind on the right path because it is now metamorphosing its habits. When this is done, our thoughts naturally do not go astray." (see source 29 p. 336)

Addressing the theory of meditation may perhaps bring comprehension, but not spiritual development. Therefore, Babuji urges everyone to try the system in practice themselves:

"I do not want you to dwell in an imagination that if you repeatedly read the scriptures you will become the master of spirituality. By so doing you can become a philosopher or learned man, but you cannot be a yogi without actual practice with love and devotion. It is very difficult to put a practical thing in words, just as you cannot describe the taste of wheat although you have eaten it many a time." ...

"I have shown the efficacy of Raja Yoga. It is the only thing which can weave one's destiny. It is complete in itself. Practice and anubhava [intuitive experience] only can reveal it. I do not ask you to believe me blindly, but I would most solemnly request you to practice it in right earnest and see that things are coming to your knowledge. There are other methods too to practise Raja Yoga; but I assure you this method, as given in this book [source 30], is the most benefiting. My sincere advice to the readers is to seek the adept in this science. It is very difficult to find such a person, but they are there, no doubt, in this world." (see source 30 p. 171 and p. 165-166)

Constant Remembrance – a "Shortcut"

Being in remembrance of the divine all the time in everything you do is called *Constant Remembrance* in Sahaj Marg. When you connect to the Master who has attained the highest spiritual state, realisation, this will also connect you to the divine essence in which He is absorbed.

How this is possible, that the heart's capacity can be refined with Constant Remembrance so that it is able to embrace the divine essence, cannot be described in words. The process takes place in the field outside the intellect's framework of comprehension. Therefore, I would recommend that throughout this chapter you, as the reader, allow your heart to sense what words can't describe so that you also intuitively perceive the essence of the concept of Constant Remembrance.

It is difficult for us human beings to maintain our focus on the abstract omnipresent divine state. Most people will find it easier to connect themselves with the divine state through love for a Master in human form. Through Constant Remembrance the student develops love for the Master. Only with a devoted and loving heart can the student forget "himself/herself" and become one with the divine state. It is necessary with an unconditional love for the Master in order to achieve realisation.

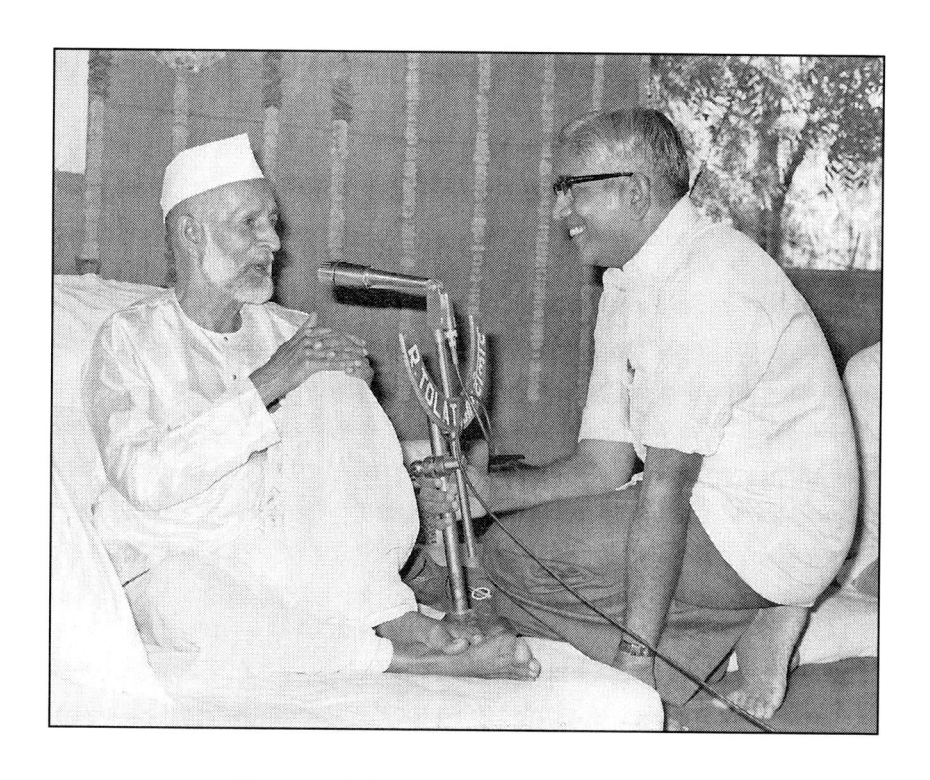

Chariji with his Master Babuji. See source IX

There are several ways to be in Constance Remembrance with the Master – these among others: you can either recall the physical picture of the Master internally in order to recall the connection, or you can focus on the feeling of connection with the Master in your heart and keep your attention on this contact.

Attainment of realisation through Constant Remembrance can only be done when the Master himself has achieved realisation and has thus become a personification of the divine essence. The concept of Constant Remembrance can, therefore, be expressed as "constantly being in remembrance of the Master" and thus at one with his inner spiritual state and capacity. Keeping focus on the Master, 24 hours a day, 7 days a week, will therefore be the ultimately fastest road to achieving the goal for spiritual development. Therefore, Constant Remembrance constitutes a "shortcut" to realization.

The reason that the Master is a crucial link to God is explained by Babuji as follows:

"It is only the helping support of a capable guide that can take us on up to our destination." ...

"The help of a Guru or Master is, therefore, essential and indispensable for those engaged in spiritual pursuit. There have been cases, however, where sages have attained perfection by mere selfeffort, surrendering themselves direct to God. But such examples are rare. It is really a very difficult course and can be followed only by persons, specially gifted with uncommon genius. Guru is the connecting link between God and man. It is through his medium only that we can reach God. He is the only power that can extricate us from the intricacies of the Path." (see source 31 pp. 43 and 44)

The explanation for the importance of using Constant Remembrance is that we develop love through Constant Remembrance – and it is love that leads us all the way to realisation. Chariji explains this as follows:

"Babuji has said, "If you are able to remember the Master continuously, constantly, the need for meditation drops off." Why? Here is the great difference between most of the yogic systems and ours. Because here the foundation of a spiritual association with the Master is love. And to create love there is no other way but constant remembrance." (see source 36 p. 51)

"If there is Love, you don't need anything else. If not, you need tolerance, you need faith, you need courage, and you must not have prejudices." (see source 47 p. 10)

The reason that you can develop love for the Master through Constant Remembrance is this: Normally, you automatically remember the one you love ... Conversely, if you choose to think of someone constantly, you will "automatically" develop love for this person. When you think constantly of the Master, you will come to love him, and if you love the Master completely and wholly, you are one with Him – and thus one with his state. This is why the Master constitutes an instrument for us to open and develop love in our hearts and through this connect to the divine essence which He represents. Once this connection is established, the goal is achieved; we will be fused together with the divine essence and permanently bound to it. Chariji expresses this as follows:

"But constant remembrance too is only a process. For what? To develop love for the Master. Because it is a technique. When we love, we remember those whom we love. Reverse the process. Remember him and you begin to love him. Now when you start loving him, remembrance automatically, as a process, stops. Because you love and you remember automatically." ...

""... Put Him inside yourself in your heart." In fact, He is there already. Recognise His presence and feed yourself to Him, by thinking of Him constantly.

So the exercise to think of Him constantly is what we try to achieve by thinking of Him occasionally in meditation." (see source 40 p. 123 and source 39 p. 53)

When, as a student, you connect in Constant Remembrance with Chariji and thus with his inner state, you connect at the same time with Babuji, Lalaji and the divine essence. The reason is that all three Masters have achieved realisation, so their state is identical and also at one with the divine state. Lalaji achieved realisation by himself in just seven months. Babuji achieved realisation with the help of his Master, Lalaji. In the process Babuji developed complete devotion to Lalaji, and gave him the credit for everything which he himself was able to accomplish. In the same way Babuji supported Chariji in becoming a Master and Chariji developed the same complete devotion towards Babuji. Similarly, Chariji gives Babuji "the credit for everything – all his abilities, skills and everything he is able to achieve. When none of these Masters take credit themselves for what they can do and are, they avoid building ego and karma. Thus their state remains one with their

Masters" state and as such pure and free from ego tendencies. In the same way students today can achieve this pure state through love and devotion to Chariji – through Constant Remembrance.

Babuji explains the practical execution of Constant Remembrance and its beneficial effect:

"We must feel ourselves connected with the Supreme Power every moment with an unbroken chain of thought during all our activities. It can be easily accomplished if we treat all our action and work to be a part of divine duty, entrusted to us by the Great Master [God] whom we are to serve as best as we can. Service and sacrifice are the two main instruments with which we build the temple of spirituality, love of course being the fundamental basis." ...

"If you cultivate this feeling and maintain the outlook that your Master is doing everything in your place, you shall not only be in constant remembrance all the while, but your action will cause no impression whatsoever and very soon you will cease making further samskaras [samskaras are the after effects of impressions which create karma which have to be phased out later on]." (see source 31 p. 80-81 and p. 84)

In the above quotation Babuji mentions that when you live in Constant Remembrance, you stop creating samskara – after – effects of impressions that are stored in the mind. This is an extremely crucial gain on the spiritual path, because the mind does not become completely "clean" until the moment all old samskara is dissolved. During our everyday lives we are all exposed to impressions. The after-effects of these impressions are new samskara which are added to the heap of the previous ones. In this way our burden of samskara grows. Because you do not add new samskara to the collection when in Constant Remembrance, all your samskara can quickly be dissolved and the mind become "clean". This is a necessary result which we all must attain in order to be able to reach higher stages on our path of spiritual development.

When you are able to live in Constant Remembrance, then you no longer need to practise meditation. Then contact with the divine state is permanent. You forget yourself and choose to live in the light of His light. Chariji describes this as follows:

"So that is the potential, I should say infinite potency, of the remembrance process. It begins to breed love in your heart for the one you remember. Then the whole goal is, I mean it is there before you, you don't have to reach anything any more. As Babuji said, "Love Him in such a way that your love knocks on His heart so that He has to open the door and come out and sees who is there. Then your job is done."" ...

"Therefore constant remembrance too is a process and so meditation goes, constant remembrance goes. Now love remains. When love remains, where is the question of getting, becoming, associating, all this nonsense, you see? That is still because we think of him and me as two separate entities. Therefore merger is the final result, where I have forgotten myself in his existence. I don't exist, He exists." (see source 40 p. 125 and p. 124)

"We must be very careful that we don't ask our Master for gifts of power, gifts of happiness, but we ask Him for Himself. Only Love can make this possible." ...

"And if and when this third stage [when Constant Remembrance has progressed to at stage of love for the Master] *is achieved, our work more or less is finished. Because, as Babuji explained, the beloved now begins to remember the lover. Our love knocks on His heart, and when His heart opens to our love, our work is over. And as Babuji repeated so many times, that is where spirituality really begins."* ...

"My Master says, if God gives you the entire universe, it is still at waste unless He comes with you." (see source 42 ppp. 14, 13-14, 14)

"That is why he [Babuji] *also says constant remembrance is only a technique, and when you, through your love, have given me permanent residence in*

your heart, remembrance goes. Not in the sense that we forget, but the need to remember is gone, because He is my Self." (see source 32 p. 219-220)

Only God – in the form of the highest state – is able to be in all places at all times and thus able to be present completely and fully with all people at any time. Therefore, Constant Remembrance only works when it is God that we are in remembrance of, and therefore the Master must be one with the divine state. For when you think of one of your own loved ones, they are not automatically with you – only God will be with you always. Chariji expresses this as follows:

"So it is only God whom you can remember, everyone of us can remember, all over the world, everywhere, and who can respond to that call of your remembrance instantly, and yet He is there too, wherever He may be, wherever He is seated, you see. Therfore the need to love God, love the Master." (see source 40 p. 139)

Description of the divine state

The divine state – the actual goal of spiritual development – is described by Babuji as follows:

"Reality is not a thing to be perceived through physical organs of sense but it can only be realized in the innermost core of the heart."

"The final point of approach is where every kind of force, power, activity or even stimulus disappears and a man enters a state of complete negation, Nothingness or Zero. That is the highest point of approach or the final goal of life." ...

"Most of the scholarly saints have defined the state of realization in numerous odd ways, but to me it appears that so far as it can be defined, it is not realization. It is really a dumb state which is beyond expression.

Feeling or observing luminosity within or outside is not realization at all. During the early period of my abhyas, I often felt and witnessed luminosity. But that not being the goal, I proceeded on under the watchful support of my master. Really it is a tasteless state-unchanging and constant. There is no charm, no attraction, and no "anandam" [bliss] *in the popular sense of the word. It can more appropriately be described as "sang-e-benamak" (i.e., a lump of salt from which saltishness has been taken away). One having attained the state of realization develops an unfailing will in the spiritual sphere."* (see source 31 p. 91 and p. 24-25 and source 29 p. 323-324)

Is it necessary to have a spiritual Master?

As previously mentioned, the earth is now in the era called kaliyuga – the age of darkness. That we in our time need outside help in order to become aware of the light in our hearts and make it shine, is explained by Babuji in the following way where he also gives the reason for Lalaji's birth:

"Great men are not accidentally born, but when the time needs them most they come, do their job and go – such is the phenomenon of nature. India, which has always been the home of spirituality, was groping in darkness and had totally forgotten the age-old system of yoga. Solid materialism had taken the place of fine spiritualism. Dark clouds of ignorance were hovering all over. Yogic transmission had become quite foreign to the Hindus. At this stage, when spirituality was tottering helplessly, some great Personality was urgently needed to set things right for the uplift of mankind.

At such a time the power of Nature descended in human form as Samarth Guru Mahatma Ram Chandraji Maharaj [Lalaji from Fathegarh], at Farrukhabad the district (U.P.) [North India]." (see source 30 p. 119)

Babuji's argument as to why a guru is necessary on the spiritual path and also his reassuring words that you can always drop the guru again, are as follows:

"What we stand in need of from a guru is the true impulse to effect the awakening of the soul and his direct support in the course of our further march on the path of realization. Such a man we have to seek for, if we aim at success." ...

"God is the real Guru or Master and we get Light from Him alone. But as it is extremely difficult for a man of ordinary talents to draw inspiration from God direct, we seek the help of one of our fellow beings who has established his connection with the Almighty." ...

"The need of a guru or master, grows greater and greater as we go on advancing and securing higher stages. Books are of no avail to us in this respect." ...

"Actual realization comes only after training in the realm of practice, and for that, knowledge or erudition proves to be of little assistance. The help of a guru or master is, therefore, essential and indispensable for those engaged in spiritual pursuit." ...

"Hence we must connect ourselves with such a great power by feelings of love and attraction. It does not matter much what conception of him we entertain in our mind. We may call him our friend, Master, servant or whatever we might be pleased to choose. But he remains after all our guide or guru, as he is commonly called." ...

"I hold it to be the birthright of every man to break off from his guru at any time if he finds that he had made a wrong selection or had misjudged the guru's capacity or worth. He is also free to seek another guru if at any stage he finds that his guru has not the capacity to take him beyond what he has already acquired." (See source 31 p. 51, p. 56-57, pppp. 43 and 44 and 45 and 48)

Chariji often uses the following this image to illustrate the need for a Master: A guru is like a mountain guide who can support the inexperienced climbers who want to reach the top of the mountain. There are many chasms and rough ground on the way up. But he who has trod this path knows where there are footholds and the direction for the next step. On this trip you need to have complete trust in your mountain guide. His instructions must be followed without hesitation if you are to reach the top. Therefore, every person who wishes to climb must weigh the mountain guide candidates carefully on a golden scales. The final choice must not be made until he or she feels absolutely convinced that the leader in question is the greatest capacity in the field. Besides having the ability to lead others on the right path, a true Master must also be able to transform the path itself – from being a difficult path to becoming a very easy path. Chariji explains this in the following way:

"... if you are really trying for the high ranges and the highest ranges and to reach the peak, of course you know, very soon there is hardly a way. You have to find it. That is why mountaineers have guides, whether in Switzerland or in the Himalayas or in the Andes. Nobody would imagine or be foolish enough to try to climb without a guide in front of him, because the guide knows the way, though there is no visible way. You look and look and look, and there is no way you see, and then amazingly, this guide, he ties himself to you risking being pulled down by you too. His life is in your hands. Because if there is a crazy fellow climbing behind who loses confidence, or who does not trust the guide at a particular moment, he may panic, and if he falls the guide has to fall with him, there is no other way, you see." ...

"Now, similarly, what you need when you want to climb the spiritual mountain is a great deal of courage that you must reach the top, even if you are going to die in the process. Those who are not willing to die in the process will hardly ever make it. But it is a strange thing that one who is willing to die rarely dies, and one who wants to avoid death is risking death every second. So we must be prepared. Well, there is no toe hold, there is no finger hold, except that fellow going up in front of me; and he looks so skinny, and he doesn't seem to have bathed for three days and he speaks some sort of a patois, which I don't understand. Well, just follow him. He is not giving you instructions. He says, I have tied you to myself, follow." ...

"People behind are thinking, "What is this? They are going so easily up this mountain. What is this miracle?" And somebody shouts, "Hello," and you say, "Yes?" "How do you climb that mountain?" We say, "It's very easy. There is no mountain to climb. It appears to you like a mountain from there. Come here, and see the miracle that it is still a mountain but it is no longer a mountain." So that is the guidance of the Master you see, that he transforms an increasingly difficult path into an increasingly easier path, so that at the most difficult stretches, it is as if we are just floating on air and going through that piece. So, why I say this, we should not worry that the path seems to be difficult. Because not only is the Master in Sahaj Marg a guide, he is not only a mountain guide, tying himself to you and risking his life for your sake, and pulling you sometimes, pushing you sometimes, cursing you sometimes. He is the Master who changes the way itself into something easy. So that is the sort of guidance and help that we get in Sahaj Marg." (See source 40 pp. 51 and 52-53 and 56)

Babuji compares the task of a true Master in relation to his students with the role of a mother's relationship with her child – and therefore it would further the student's relationship with the Master if the student regards him as a spiritual mother:

"The function of a mother and of a true guru are closely similar. The mother retains a child within her womb for a certain duration. The guru too retains the spiritual child within his mental sphere for a certain duration. During this period the disciple, like the baby in the womb, sucks energy and gets nourishment from the spiritual waves of the guru's thoughts. When the time matures, he is born in a brighter world and thence his own spiritual life begins. If the disciple enters the mental sphere of the guru surrendering all belongings to him, it takes only seven months to deliver him into the brighter world. But the process is generally delayed for a considerable time because while living in the guru's mental sphere the disciple retains the consciousness of his own thoughts and feelings. Thus we find that the position of a guru is much the same as that of a mother. The conception of guru as a spiritual mother promotes in us feelings of love, reverence and surrender which are the main factors of spiritual life." (see source 29 p. 349-350)

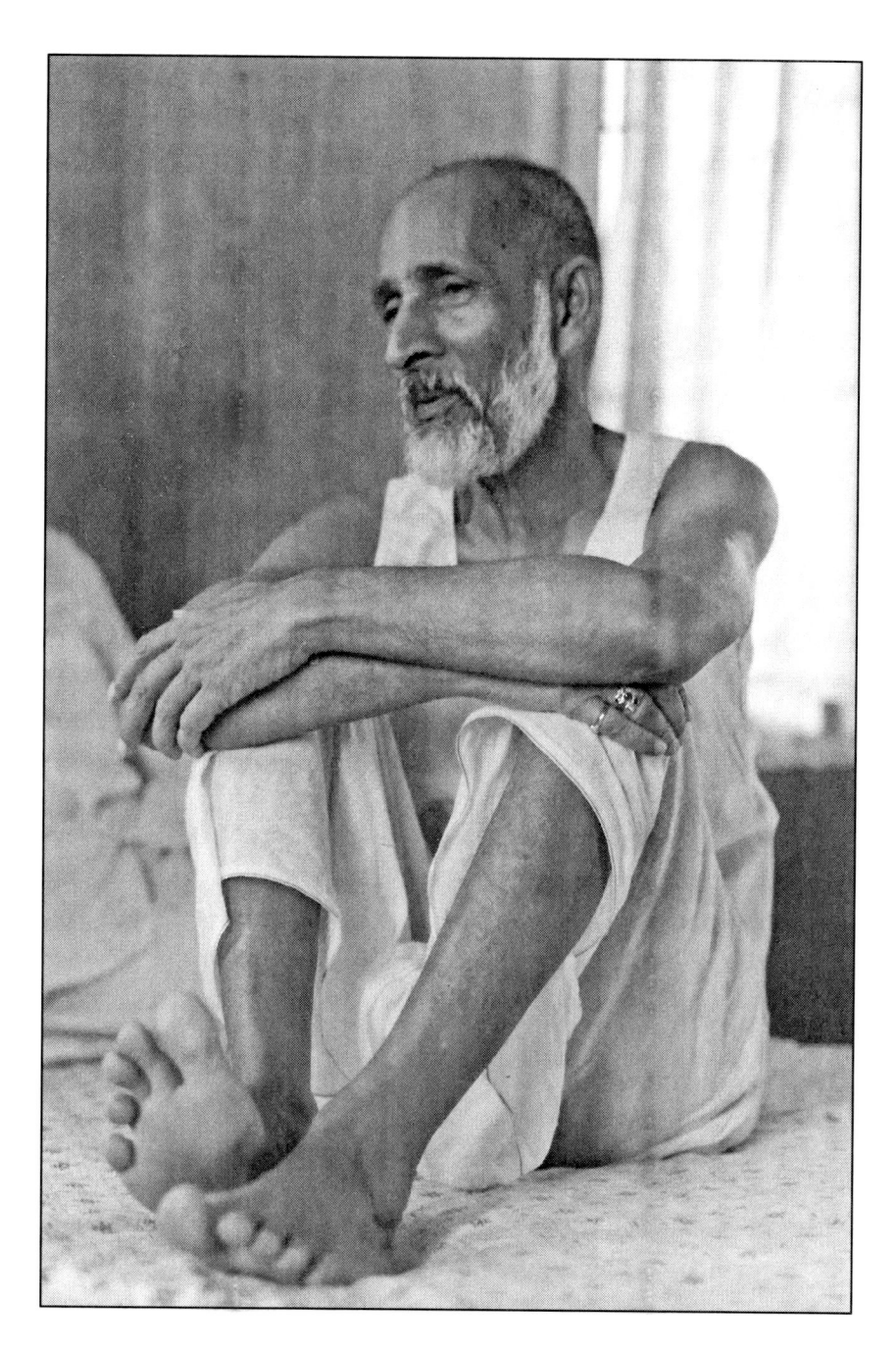

Babuji. See source IX

Some people may feel resistance against surrendering themselves to a spiritual Master. Chariji points out that surrender is a relatively logical and simple approach which we use in other connections in our lives. He refers to the following example which Babuji once gave as an answer to the same question:

"Once Master [Babuji] clarified this point with a third illustration. What do we do when we go to a doctor for treatment? We accept all that he says. We abide by his regimen of diet and medication. We follow his precription on what we are to do and what we are to abstain from doing. If surgery is necessary we allow ourselves to be anaesthetised into a totally inactive condition so as to permit him to operate upon us. We have to do all this if the doctor is to succeed in helping us. Does this not imply a surrender to the doctor's will and method? Can we question his method? Can we ask for a guarantee of success? Yet without all this we are prepared to surrender ourselves to the will of the doctor. Why, then, cannot we duplicate this attitude in our spiritual life? In spiritual life we ask for proofs first – proof of the existence of God, let us say; proof of the system's efficacy, and so on. Master said this was not only wrong but illogical. Master added, "Suppose I am willing to offer proof, how many can understand the proof? Look here, suppose you ask a scientist to prove certain abstract ideas, how many can understand the proof? And the higher the work the more difficult it is to understand the subject. So we should try the system, and our own experience of the work will furnish the proof from within ourselves."" (see source 37 p. 34-35)

When is a guru a true Master?

As mentioned, being a guru means just being a teacher. So the designation is no guarantee for the teacher's capacity or competence. The same rules apply to spirituality as to other fields. In order to really be able to assess the full capacity of a guru, you have to be a guru yourself. Therefore, I will not attempt to explain anything about this, but leave it to Babuji instead. Via the following quotations he gives guidelines for the qualities which – in his opinion – a true Master must possess.

Babuji's characterisation of a guru and the requirements to his abilities are as follows:

"A guru must, therefore, necessarily be quite devoid of any personal motive or selfish interest. He must be totally free from all feelings of pride or greatness. He must be a selfless man and a true servant of humanity at large, teaching people out of pure love without any ulterior selfish motive of name, fame or money. He must have his access up to the farthest possible limit and must have the power of yogic transmission. Such a man we must seek for as our guide if we want complete success. It is better to remain without a guru all our life than to submit to the guidance of an unworthy guru." …

"The popular meaning of a mahatma [a great soul] *as a great individual does not appeal to me. I would define a mahatma as the most insignificant being or rather a neglected figure, beyond all feelings of greatness, pride or egoism, dwelling permanently in a state of complete self-negation."* (see source 31 p. 59 and source 29 p. 357)

Babuji describes a method of assessing a true Master based on the feelings which his nearness arouses in a person's body and mind and not the least, within his or her heart:

"I tell you an easy method of finding them out [the true masters]. If you sit beside such a person, never mind be he a sannyasi [one who has renounced worldly life and leads a secluded life] or a grihastha [one who lives a worldly family life], calmness, the nature of self, will remain predominant and you will be carefree for the time being. You will remain in touch with the Real thing so long as you are with him. The effect is automatic, i.e., even if he does not exert himself. So if you really want to search for such a person, what you have to do is only to look to your own heart and note

the condition of your mind. It becomes comparatively calm and quiet, and the different ideas that have been haunting your mind and troubling you all the time are away so long as you are with him. But one thing is to be clearly borne in mind, that mind should not in any way be taxed and there should be no heaviness. Because this effect (keeping off the ideas and bringing the working of the mind to a standstilll) can be brought forth also by those who have mastered the baser sciences, e.g., mesmerism and hypnotism, et cetera. But the difference between the two is that in the latter case heaviness, exhaustion and dullness of the mind and physique will be felt, while in the former case the person will feel lightness and at the same time calmness shall be prevailing all over. It is just possible that you may not be able to judge it at the first glance, but constant company with the person will surely offer you clear hints and indications in this respect." (see source 30 p. 166)

The decisive difference between the theorists and the true Masters whose knowledge is based on their own experience is illustrated by Babuji in the following quotations. He emphasises that a prerequisite for attaining realisation is that the soul is awakened in the heart. A true Master can do this for his students – a task which lies outside the framework of theoretical knowledge. Therefore, only a Master who has attained realisation himself can support students on their path of spiritual development.

"It must well be borne in mind that it is not the learning or knowledge that makes a man perfect but it is only realization in the right sense that makes a true yogi or saint ... Similarly the real test of a mahatma or guru is not his miracles but experience on the path of realization ... There are some who hold the view that knowledge being the preliminary stage of realization is essential and indispensable. I do not agree with them on the grounds that knowledge is only an achievement of the brain, whereas realization is the awakening of the soul; and hence, far beyond its scope. Therefore a real teacher is not one who can explain to us the soundness of the religious dogmas or who can prescribe to us do's and don'ts. What we stand in need from a guru is the true impulse to effect the awakening of

the soul, and his direct support in the course of our further march on the path of realization. Such a man we have to seek for, if we aim at success ... A man who is himself free can free you from eternal bondage." (see source 29 p. 356-357)

"The solution of the problem as to what sort of man should be selected as a guide or guru is not difficult to seek. When our eyes are fixed on the final goal we can never be satisfied with any one who appears to be short of the mark. Every saint or yogi has got his own level of attainment and of self-elevation. If we attach ourselves with any one of them with faith and devotion and secure merging with his highest condition, we will ourselves attain corresponding elevation. It is, therefore, absolutely necessary to select one of the highest attainments as our guru. If unfortunately we are somehow or other induced to select one of inferior attainments we will correspondingly be lagging behind in our final approach." (see source 31 p. 55-56)

Babuji illustrates below why it is crucial to choose a guru who possesses the capacity to transmit. He illustrates what transmission is and what a unique help a Master can accomplish for his student:

"Here I may assure you that spiritual training for the attainment of higher stages is only possible by the process of yogic transmission and by no other means."

"It is a great wonder when a great personality like Lord Krishna, Swami Vivekananda or my Master changes the entire course of a man's life. It is absolutely necessary for us to find out such a guide who can lift us higher and higher by his power. This mystery is known as "pranahuti" – the power of transmission. This is power working through the channels of pure mind. Pranahuti is effected through the power of will which is always effective. If a trainer in spirituality exerts his will to mould the mind of the trainee, it will be effective and yield excellent results." ...

"... the power of transmission is a yogic attainment of a very high order by which a yogi can infuse by his will-force the yogic energy or Godly effulgence within any one, and remove anything unwanted in him or detrimental to his spiritual progress. He can exercise this power not only on those assembled around him, but on those too, who are away from him. The power can be utilised in any way or at any time. One who has got command over this power can, at a glance, create temporarily or permanently, a condition of mind which is far ahead of the existing condition of the mind of the abhyasi, and which, otherwise, will require a lifetime to be achieved ... Sages have often, through power of transmission, changed the entire nature of a man at a mere glance. The wonderful examples of the great sages like my master Samarth Guru Mahatma Rma Chandraji Maharaj of Fatehgarh [Lalaji], Swami Vivekananda and others offer ample proof of it." (see source 31 p. 53 and source 29 pp. 358 and 361-362)

Babuji warns against the fact that some gurus profess to be able to transmit, while this in actual fact is not the case. You may believe erroneously that transmission is happening, when in actual fact it is just the natural charisma from these people which is affecting people around them. It is important to observe what is happening in the mind when one is with a guru. The natural charisma only gives a short-term impact, while transmission has a permanent effect.:

"It generally happens that when you are in the company of a mahatma or a saint, you are to some extent relieved of your disturbing thoughts and feel comparatively calm for a while. This they claim to be due to the effect of transmission by the mahatma. Those who offer this explanation, mean only to deceive the public with a view to whitewashing their incapacity.

What they interpret as transmission is really the automatic radiation of the pious "paramanus" (fine particles) from the mahatma. It affects all those assembled there with the result that calmness prevails to some extent, so long as they are there. It is only a natural process and has nothing to do with transmission. It is not only from a mahatma or saint that such "paramanus" (fine particles) radiate, but also from everyone whether pious or wicked, saintly or devilish. If you are for some time with an impious or morally degraded person, you find impious "paramanus" radiating from him and affecting you, with the result that you find your thoughts flowing in the same channel for the time being.

The effect of such radiation remains only for a little while and disappears when you are away from it." (see source 29 p. 360-361)

Babuji continues by warning about other methods used by false prophets; among others, those who perform so-called miracles in order to attract students in this way.

"A raja yogi endowed with the power of transmission can no doubt display miracles but he never likes to do so since that will be derogatory to his real conditions. We have the example of Christ who displayed miracles all his life. But in spite of all that, he got only twelve disciples among whom there was even that one who subsequently brought about his crucifixion. That shows that his miracles were of no avail in promoting faith among people. It was, in fact, his noble teachings alone that afterwards secured for him such a large following. It is, therefore, in our best interest, to have our eyes fixed upon Reality rather than upon miracles which are undoubtedly very petty affairs and can be displayed by a person of comparatively inferior attainments and talents. Miracles are no criterion for a saint or a yogi. It is, on the other hand, a deliberate fraud played by dexterous gurus upon weak and credulous people to entrap them in the fold of their gurudom. Before deciding about the final selection, one must be fully convinced of a man's capabilities and merits with regard to his practical attainments on the path. For this he must have continued association with him to judge things through perceptions and experience in a practical way. When he is thus convinced, he must then trust him in good faith and rely upon him firmly. This is very essential for a successful pursuit." (see source 29 p. 350-351)

Some gurus call themselves avatars. Therefore, I will let Babuji's description of the special characteristics of avatars conclude this chapter on assessing gurus. In the last quotation Babuji refers to the power of the "Root". It is my understanding, that the Root must be the essence from which our universe was created.

"The avatars come down for a definite purpose, endowed with all the necessary powers required for the accomplishment of the work, allotted to them. That may, in other words, serve to be their samskaras which brought them down into the world. The power withdraws them after their work is finished. The difference between an ordinary man and an avatar is that man is covered with numerous sheets while an avatar is free from most of them. They have the Divine within their perception, while a man is deprived of it. Now though the origin of man and avatar is the same, the avatar is in closer contact with the Divine. Everything he stands in need of, comes to him from the eternal store. He receives divine commands to guide him in his works which are popularly known as divine inspirations (deva-vani)." ...

"None of the avatars who so far came down to the earth had ever been bestowed with the power of the Root. I give this out on the basis of my reading of Nature through the kind grace of God who alone is the real knower of things." (see source 29 pp. 311-312 and 312)

How do you find "Your Master"?

Making contact with the Master who can help you develop on the spiritual path is a responsibility that rests on both the aspirant and the Master. Chariji describes this as follows:

"One of the roles of a true guru would therefore appear to be that of awaiting the call of a devoted heart, and responding to it. When one goes deeper into this matter, one finds that even this is a superficial view. What really happens is that Master "prepares the field," as he puts it, by continued

work of a spiritual nature. Receptive souls are attracted towards him, and the contact becomes a direct spiritual contact. It would be appropriate to say that the aspirant, ready for the spiritual path, waits at home in a prayerful attitude inviting the guru to come to him. This is the simplest and the best way, as one can rarely know even where to seek the guru, should one set out on at journey to seek him. "All things come to him who waits," says an old proverb, and this applies most pertinently to the coming of a guru into a person's life. The guru, on his part, is putting out spiritual feelers, as it were, and when the feeler finds a perceptive person there is information fed back to the guru. He then commences the prepartation of the abhyasi forthwith, by transmission. Physical contact between the guru and the disciple may come very much later. The exact time of occurrence of the personal relationship is unimportant in so far as the abhyasi's preparation is concerned." (see source 37 p. 125-126)

Chariji quotes Babuji's answer to the same question as follows:

*"The real search should be an inner search. A person may go from place to place all over the world, spending his whole life-time, and yet not succeed in finding a guru. The mistake we make is in looking, or searching for a guru. The right way is to **pray** for a guru. What should we do? We should pray direct to God, with deep longing in our hearts, that He may send us a worthy guide. And when we are ready for him the guru will himself knock on our door."* (see source 37 p. 124)

Why only one Master?

When I was travelling round to the four different gurus in 1994, I met the same attitude over and over again: that one should have only one Master and not "shop around" from one to another. This was a source of frustration for me, because in fact I felt the need to take a good look at the various gurus. One of the best explanations for the idea of just having one Master is the following: If you want to cross a river, there may be many boats by the banks which can all take you across to the other side. But if you try to cross the river with a leg in each boat, you will never get to the other bank.

I will let Chariji answer this question about only one guru below. He points out partly that the necessary energy is only obtained by focussing on one thing at a time, and partly that a heart can only be given fully to one person:

"... [in this excerpt, Chariji starts by referring to a statement by Babuji:] "... if at one time you are trying to achieve fifty different objectives, your mind's power is divided into fifty different channels. Therefore we have to try to achieve one thing at a time." I think there is an ancient proverb, "One thing at a time and that done well." One thing at a time and we are able to do it well. If you are trying to do twenty things, nothing gets done. Therefore he [Babuji] said, "Have one Goal, have one method, and stick to one Master, and you can achieve something." If you try to mix several things, like using one God in another method in another way, nothing is achieved. So I think it is a great piece of wisdom that he [Babuji] took meditation on light in the heart, divine light in the heart, because it makes it possible for all of us to follow it without any crisis of conscience, and achieve the final Goal." (see source 39 p. 213)

"So you see this is the secret of love. And this is what we are dealing with in spirituality. This is the sort of love we talk about when we say, "Having given, you cannot give again." This is the sort of morality of which we speak, that having given once to someone, you cannot give it to somebody else again. It is not something you can deal with as if it is a thing, you see, to be broken up and divided. A heart is given whole or not at all. It cannot be cut up into pieces, a hundred and two pieces to be distributed to a hundred and two different individuals. It cannot be even given piece by piece to one person and claimed that this is morality, because I've only given it to the same person. It is given once, wholly, or not at all." (see source 38 p. 54)

Prayer – to whom and for what?

As mentioned, a special prayer is part of the daily practice of Sahaj Marg. You say it within yourself in the evening at bedtime where you also meditate on it for a few minutes. In the morning you repeat it once as an introduction to the meditation. Chariji writes about the prayer:

"Prayer remains the most important and unfailing means of success." (see source 44 p. 32)

The prayer in Sahaj Marg was dictated word for word to Babuji by Lalaji after the latter had left his physical body. It is of utmost importance that the prayer is recited with these exact words. This is the original wording:

"O, Master!
Thou art the real goal of human life.
We are yet but slaves of wishes,
Putting bar to our advancement.
Thou art the only God and Power,
To bring us up to that Stage."
(see source 34 p. 32)

The prayer is not "asking for something", but instead an *ascertainment* of the state of things. In the prayer we state, where we are on our path, what is holding us back and what can help us to move on. Regarding the ideal way of praying Babuji writes, among other things, as follows: that it is important to prepare your inner state for prayer so that in prayer you are able first to present God with your true state and thereafter submit completely to His will. The greatest effect is achieved in this manner:

"... the most important and unfailing means of success is the prayer. It connects our link with God to whom we surrender ourselves with love and devotion. In prayer we stand before Him as a humble suppliant presenting

to Him our true state and completely resigning ourselves to His will. This is the true form of prayer and as true devotees we must also feel satisfied with the Will of the Master. It is a folly to pray to God for petty wordly ends except in most exceptional cases when peace of mind is greatly disturbed for want of bare necessities. We should always pray to the supreme Master the Omnipotent and the Omniscient alone with a mind totally absorbed in love and submission to Him forgetting even ourselves altogether. This is the proper way of offering prayer which in such a state seldom goes unrewarded." (see source 31 p. 41-42)

You see that the prayer in Sahaj Marg starts with the words "O Master". The fact that you do not address God directly, but the Master, has given rise to much wondering. The question of to whom a prayer should be addressed has once been answered by Chariji as follows:

"The guru is the living God. This is the concept of guru in the Hindu tradition, in what we call the "sanathana dharma" tradition, in the yogic tradition. Beyond Him there exists no God. He is not only the object of worship, He is the object of everything. Therefore, Master [Babuji] said, if at all one has to pray, and one has a Master of calibre who is serving his needs, there is some purpose in praying to that Master. You see, I was asked a question sometime last year. Babuji himself has written that ultimately He [pointing upwards] is the real Master, you see, and all the human Masters who come on this world, on this earth, are His representatives. If that is so, then why do we address the prayer, "O Master" and not "Oh God". Now today I am giving you the answer for that. Because God, it is a living God who is before you in the form of the Master; not that God is dead elsewhere, but this is an embodied flesh-and-blood divinity, you see, who can understand our needs; who can understand our temperaments; who can sympathise with us, being human himself, who can accept our failings, perhaps having failed himself in some way." ...

"God, unfortunately, or fortunately, for us, has no mind. This is the great teaching of my Master. God cannot possibly have a mind because, if there is a mind, there is consciousness. If there is consciousness, there is consciousness of good and bad, of life and death, of myself and yourself. And the duality of

existence takes birth in his mind and He ceases to be God at the instant He is born. So Babuji's greatest research, I would say, is this finding that God cannot possibly have a mind. Therefore, He cannot even know He is God. How can He, therefore, answer your prayers, you see, coming back to the question of prayer. Which God? Where? How will He recognise that He is being addressed? "Oh God!" I shout in the wilderness you know. Yes, but who is to listen to me? Therefore, you know, in His ultimate mercy, compassion, He sends Himself in another way. You see how it is done! It is a miracle, it is a mystery.

Perhaps, as Babuji once told me when I asked him, "How does this happen?", he said, "You will know it on the day you achieve that state yourself."" (see source 36 pp. 46-47 and 47)

The lines in the prayer contain some rather special expressions and words. Chariji sheds light on these lines in the following quotations:

"Now I would like to say something about the Prayer too. Some people have the understanding that we are praying to God for something when we say this Prayer. But if you say it properly and think over what you are saying, you will find that it contains just three statements of fact.

The first line says: **"O Master! Thou art the real goal of human life."** *We are merely stating a fact. Here, the word "Master" refers to God, as Babuji Himself has written in His books. Master has written very clearly, "The real Master is He and He alone." I am clarifying this because some people ask: "How can we address a man as a Master or a Guru as a Master, when we are not addressing God in the Prayer?" Masters, as Babuji explained, are the Representatives of God. So, there should be no difficulty about any abhyasi* [people who practice the Sahaj Marg meditation system], *from any religious background, using this prayer for this purpose. So the first line of the Prayer really says:* **"God! You are the real goal of human life."** *And in a sense, we are reminding ourselves of what the Goal is, which we are trying to achieve.*

The second line of the prayer says: **"We are yet but slaves of wishes putting bar to our advancement."** *We are not asking God to remove the* wishes or to change our wishes or anything like that. We are again making a statement of fact. That is, we are saying, with an attitude of humility, that we recognize that we are the problem creators ourselves. We humbly state that our wishes are putting bar to our advancement. If effectively used, this prayer will prevent us from developing wishes for the future.

The third line says: **"Thou art the only God and power to bring us up to that stage."** *Here, we recognize the fact that by our own effort, nothing is possible. We are stating to ourselves the fact that He alone can help us to take us up to that stage of existence. Again, please note that we are not asking God for any help whatsoever."* ...

"So, in a relation of love between two persons, either the lover goes to the beloved or the beloved comes to the lover only, so that they can be together, not to take things away from each other. The prayer states this very beautifully because the first line says, **"Thou art the real goal,"** which means **You** are the real goal, not your powers, not your beauty, not your riches, not even the Universe, but: **You** (the beloved) are the real goal.

The last line of the prayer reaffirms this very forcibly. It says: "Only the beloved can give Himself." You cannot ask a mediator to bring the beloved to you." ...

"So the prayer consists of three statements where the first one puts before us the goal. The second one tells us what is the only impediment that is an impediment to our progress, namely our wishes, and the third one states that the goal that is God Himself has to assist us to reach Him. You will all remember that Babuji has said: "Prayer is begging." That is the traditional way of prayer, which is begging. This prayer of our Mission has no element of begging or demanding or requesting, nothing in it." ...

"We can therefore put our Mission prayer in ordinary worldly language, and say:

"My beloved, you are the real goal of my life. What is standing between us are my foolish wishes and desires for your powers, your beauty, your wealth. You alone can give me yourself."

This is all that our Mission prayer says, nothing more." (see source 42 pp. 7-8, 15, 9, 15)

My personal experience with Sahaj Marg

My personal experience as an abhyasi in Sahaj Marg is that the meditation brings me closer to my own core. When I meditate, I am taking a break from physical activities. Thus the opportunity to flee from what I do not want to be confronted with, disappears. The curtain is pulled aside in the stillness, and I must face myself and my inner state. Particularly important feelings and experiences, which I may not have noticed or have not finished with in the relevant situations, can no longer be suppressed. They come to mind where they are often followed by good ideas as to how the situations can be solved. Other times, inspiring impulses arrive out of the blue. But this thought activity is still not meditation. Not until I also let go of these thoughts and feelings can I experience just being. There are no wishes and no desires – just a sense of being which is so alluring that the daily meditation soon became a highly treasured activity for me. The effect of meditation is subtle. Slowly and little by little the personality is transformed. Sometimes I discover to my surprise that my reaction in certain situations has suddenly changed from what it was beforeThe Seminar in Denmark in 1995

without any explicable reason. Something has changed within myself without my having noticed the change. During meditation calmness of mind occurs, and the soul can have the opportunity to show itself. On days when the flow of thought seems very interesting and incessant, I can experience a feeling that this day's meditation was useless. Then I am soothed by Babuji's calming words affirming that meditation does not only have an impact on the level we are aware of, but also gives results on the unconscious level:

"The flow of ideas is due to the activities of our conscious mind which is never at rest. We are still busy in meditation with our subconscious mind, while our conscious mind is roaming about and forming numerous ideas. Thus we are not the loser in any way. In due course, after sufficient practice, the conscious mind too gets moulded and begins to act in harmony with the subconscious mind. The result thus achieved is deep-rooted and lasting, and finally calmness, the characteristic of soul becomes predominant." (see source 31 p. 68)

The Seminar in Denmark in 1995

When I at arrived at the seminar that summer, I had been practising the Sahaj Marg method for four months and was very enthusiastic. From the first day with this practice it felt right for me. The special aspect of this system was the sittings which I really felt gave me a boost when I was feeling stuck. At no time did I experience the daily practice as boring in the way that previous methods had seemed to me. All the same, I was still very uncertain of Chariji's influence on the results I achieved through my own practice and the sittings.

When I went to my first seminar in the part of Denmark called Jutland, I knew nothing of any theory about how one could assess a Master's capacity. All I had to show me the way were my experiences from India, my brain, my heart and my intuition. I would come to make diligent use of all of these.

My plan was to stay at the Jutland ashram in Vrads from 21st to 30th July 1995 while Chariji would be there. I had decided beforehand that whether or not I would continue practising Sahaj Marg would depend on my relationship with Chariji which was not yet established. Was he perhaps a mountain guide that I could trust implicitly? I aimed to find the answer in the course of this seminar.

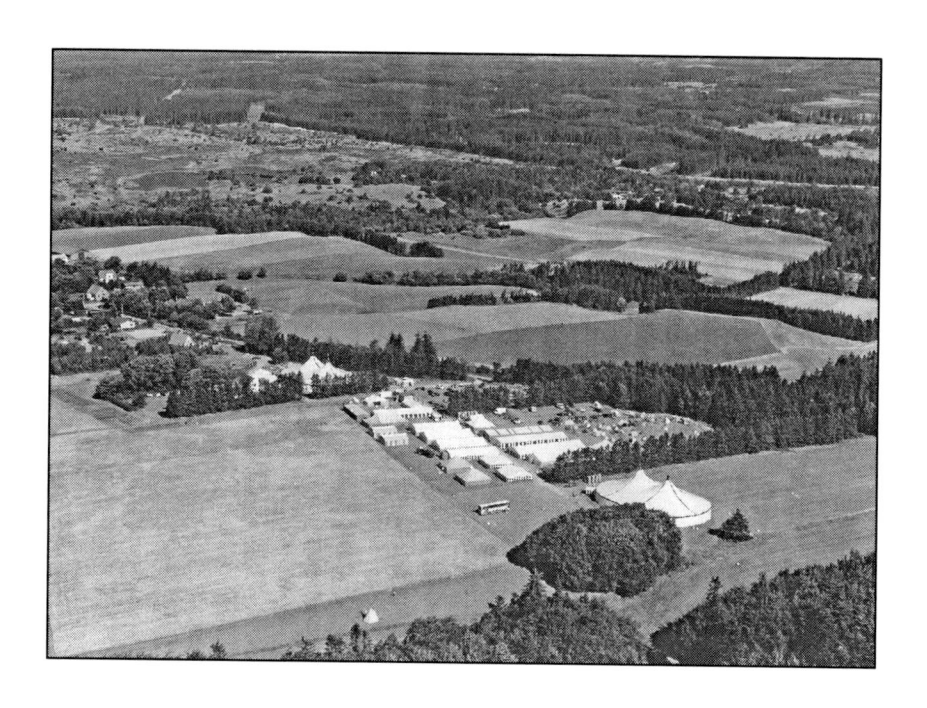

The summer seminary in Vrads 1995. The ashram can be glimpsed in the top left corner. See source X

Being with about 2,000 other participants made in itself a great impression on me. I was both surprised and overwhelmed that so many people had come from all over the world to be with Chariji here in little Denmark. Before that I had journeyed out into the world to experience something like this. Now the world was coming to me – or at least to Jutland ... There were about 200 people from Russia and others from South Africa, USA, Poland, Switzerland, England and the other European countries; there were especially many from France. There was a warmth and sense of community among the participants, regardless of their nationality. Every time I spoke to someone, I was looking into two large, sparkling eyes, radiating calm, harmony and love even though their emotions were fluctuating up and down. I had not experienced such an open and easy contact with the followers of a guru in any other ashram.

The first few days I had no direct contact with Chariji. There was nothing immediately striking about him; maybe he was just an ordinary, pleasant, elderly Indian gentleman? The only way I could see to further clarification was to study him at closer range and thus seek his physical proximity. 2-3 times a day, Chariji gave group sittings in a meditation tent where all abhyasis could be present. But because I was so intent on getting to know him better, I did not feel that the sittings were enough. In the ashram there is a small house which is Chariji's home when he visits the ashram. There is only room for specially invited abhyasis in the house. Although I did not belong to this category, I nevertheless plucked up courage to knock at the door and asked for permission to sit in his living room. I wanted to feel the energy by being like a fly on the wall. To my great surprise I was allowed to enter. This permission must be seen in the light of the fact that most of the people at a seminar like this presumably had a similar wish to get close to the Master. Of course, not everybody knocked at the door, and of those who did only a few were allowed in, so I felt myself lucky. It did not take long in the house before I reaped the fruits of my enterprise; the fly enjoyed its place on the wall. The energy around my heart began to vibrate like a song. When something feels good, you usually want more ... The rest of week I sought every opportunity to be physically close to this Master, often – but not always – with a positive result.

Whenever I was close to Chariji, I felt an inner calm and lovely sense of being. In his presence there were no questions in my mind and neither thoughts nor wishes for anything other than just *being* and resting in the group which collected around him. Everything seemed perfect to me. But when I was away from the house again and alone with myself, I kept thinking about my everyday problems, among other things a recent unhappy love affair. However, I did not feel it would be appropriate to ask Chariji for advice directly in these matters, and I did not feel the need for this at all when I was sitting opposite him. At the suggestion of other abhyasis, I wrote down my questions instead in a letter which I sent to him. I briefly outlined the four subjects which I wished to have clarified. After a couple of days I received an answer. But not in the form of a written or oral message from himself. Instead the answers came partly through words spoken to me by others and partly via a certainty which sprang up in my heart.

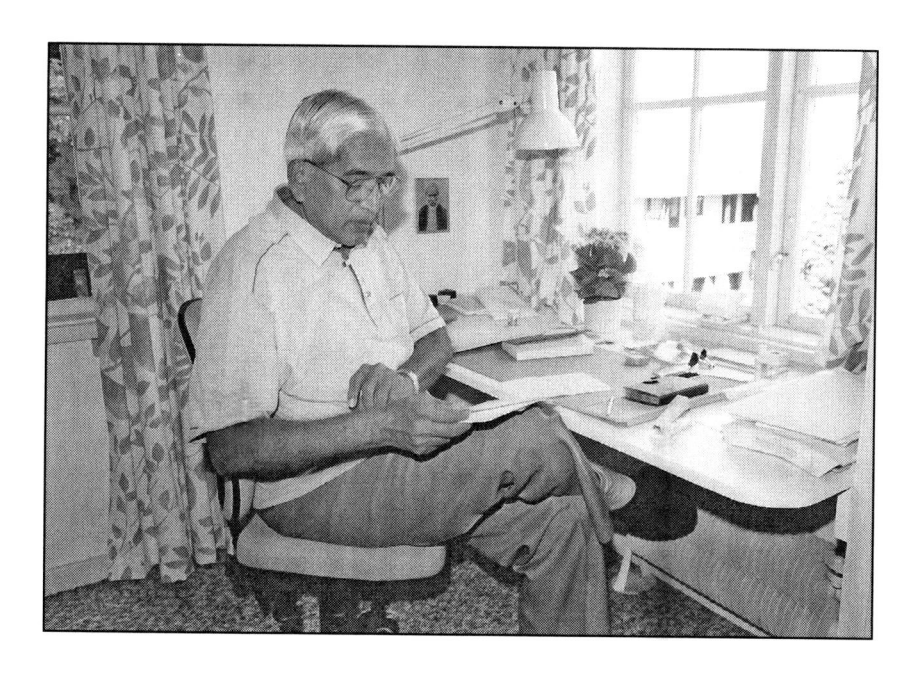

Chariji in the office of his house in the ashram in Vrads. See source X

For example, the answer to the unhappy love affair came in the following manner: An abhyasi friend came the next morning and told me that on the previous evening he had wanted to write a letter to the man involved in my unhappiness. In the letter he was going to ask the man to watch a certain film: *A Stranger Is Coming to Town*. It is about a white woman who falls in love with a black man and how her parents experience and deal with this situation. The Danish man knew about my situation which had certain similarities with the theme of the film. For I was in love with a man of Indian origin who was determined that his future wife was also to be of Indian origin. What the Danish man did not know was that the man who was involved in my unhappiness had a photo from the same film hanging on his wall – in fact this photo was the only decoration in the room. We had talked about it when I had visited him there. For him the photo represented the finest friendship that can be attained – filled with warmth and love. It was the image of the young woman's parents in the film that reflected the loving relationship between them. In view of the number of films in the world, this coincidence was rather startling. Therefore, I understood it to mean that Chariji was recommending that this relationship should just stay as a warm friendship. The wish to write the letter had arisen in the person here in Denmark at the same time as Chariji had been reading my letter that evening. This amazing coincidence convinced me that Chariji had access to other planes in the universe than the ones I knew and used.

When communicating with a Master, it is important to be aware of everything that goes on in order not to overlook the message. Even though Chariji did not answer any of the questions directly with words, I picked up and understood a lot of signals from my inner self and the people around me in the course of the seminar. Another episode which I interpreted as the answer to one of the other questions, happened like this: The following evening I was standing at the counter in the ashram café waiting for my cappuccino. When it was handed over the counter, the person on café duty accidentally knocked over a carton of milk so the contents splashed all over my body. At first I was annoyed and a little irritated at the clumsy employee. But after a while the thought came to me of how in India milk is used in ritual contexts. It is a symbol of fertility there and is poured over various symbolic figures which one wishes to bless with fertility. As one of my questions to Chariji was in fact whether I would have children in this life, I chose to interpret this milk bath as his way of showing me that I would be blessed with fertility.

After Chariji had indirectly answered all my questions in the letter, my thoughts relaxed and I had to surrender to the love that had been activated in my heart. It was as if my heart communicated with Chariji via its very own channels which I knew nothing about. My awareness had been occupied with the personal meetings with Chariji and of picking up the answers to the letter. Therefore, I was somewhat surprised one night when I could not sleep, because the same sentence kept running around in my mind in an endless repetition: In my thoughts I was telling Chariji that I surrendered to him. To put it mildly, I was amazed at this, because I had never on the journey to India in 1994 nor later ever imagined that I would "surrender" myself

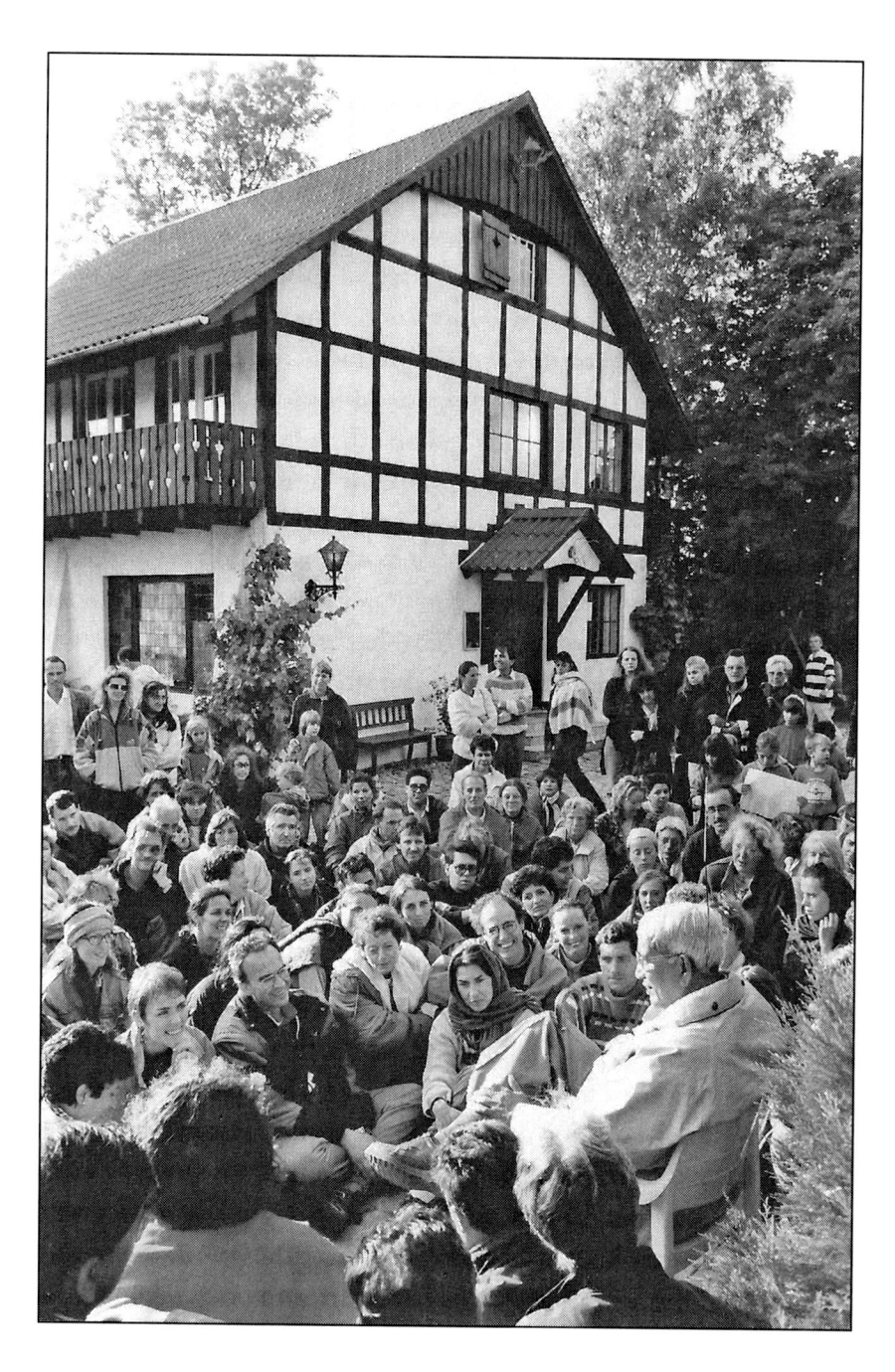

*Chariji with abhyasis by his little half-timbered
house at the ashram in Vrads. See source X*

to any Master in this way. So this thought – the strength of which was beyond compare – did not come from mental considerations, but as a message from my heart which I could not overlook. The following morning I simply had to go straight to Chariji's house and tell him that I had chosen him as my mentor. However, I was not allowed in. Luckily he came out himself soon after and I seized the opportunity to open my heart. Afterwards I had a wonderful feeling of inner liberation. I am not sure myself what this actually means. After the meeting with him, I have followed the daily practice with greater enthusiasm and have since also visited him in his Indian ashram near Chennai. In my heart I have a wonderful sensation of having come home.

Whether the help of a Master makes it easier for us ordinary people to find God in our hearts, is an open question. I personally neither can nor will ignore the attraction which my heart has towards the gurus – and in particular now to Chariji. But he can also affect my physical body. This little anecdote from the airport at Kastrup could be an indication of this:

I was out there with the other abhyasis waving goodbye when Chariji was leaving to travel on to France. When he disappeared through the passport control, I did not want to leave the airport. The others also stood around chatting for a shorter or longer time before leaving. I could neither understand nor explain my reluctance to return home. My fellow passengers from the car trip there began to be a little impatient, and I could not find any excuse for dragging out the time any more. Finally, I gave in and we started to walk towards the car. Then I remembered that I had to pay for the parking ticket inside the airport. I turned round and went back alone. On my way through the building I was suddenly taken by complete surprise. All of a sudden I was standing face to face with Chariji who gave me his hand. I understood that there were problems with his ticket and this was the reason he had to return to the check-in desk. Chariji quickly sent me on my way. I left the place filled with happiness at this surprising encounter. Perhaps he had in his own way arranged this extra goodbye, or perhaps he was welcoming me in this way. Some would say – coincidence ... well, in that case life is full of coincidences which

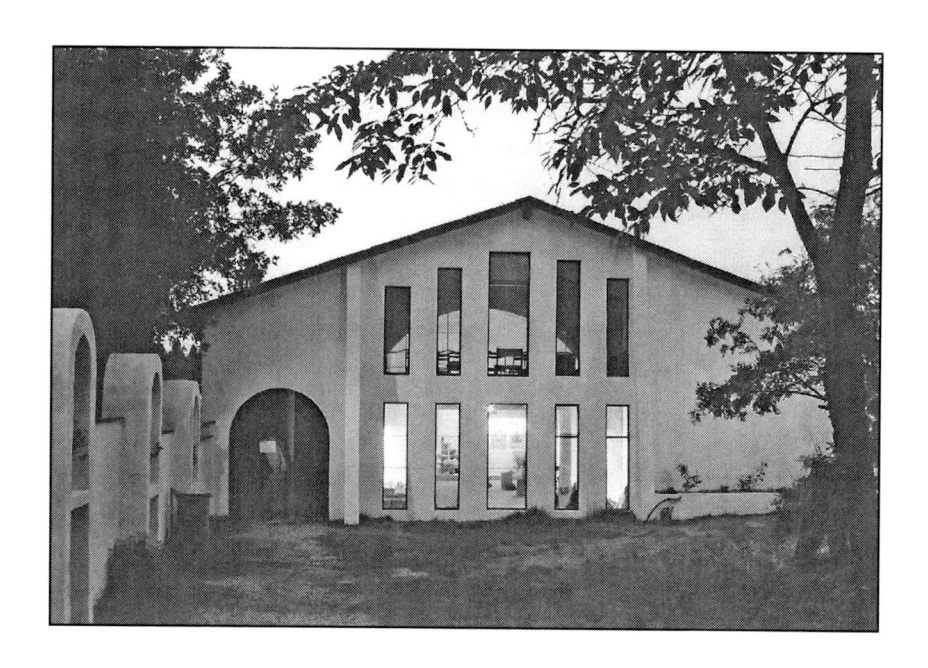

The meditation hall at the ashram in Vrads. See source X

draw perfect patterns quite by chance. When the images appear, I often discover that the coincidences might not be so coincidental after all ...

Finding the path to happiness

Travelling to India to look for gurus and palm leaf astrologers might seem like a waste of effort when I ended up by finding *the right one* in Denmark. But when the trip is so beautiful and enjoyable as my journey to India was, then it was perfectly worthwhile. And perhaps detours are unavoidable. My journey in 1994 gave me a good basis against which to measure the shortcut. As a rule you do not realise how you should have gone about something from the start until the job has been done.

The five gurus I met on my way all had the same message: that happiness is to be united with the divine in oneself; everything is in being. When we are liberated from the impressions which have imprinted themselves on the mind in this or previous lives, we become free and in harmony with the divine where the soul can expand. The path to spiritual development up the mountain is not always accessible. Sometimes one can feel afraid of plunging into the abyss. But every time a stone disappears from your back pack, it gets easier to wander on; the heavier the stone which falls, the lighter it feels afterwards.

The Master Babuji describes the goal and the steps on the way as follows:

"The highest spiritual attainment is possible only when we go beyond the limits of religion. In fact spirituality begins where religion ends. Religion is only a preliminary stage for preparing a man for his march on the path of freedom. The end of religion is the beginning of spirituality; the end of spirituality is the beginning of Reality; and the end of Reality is the real Bliss. When that too is gone, we have reached the destination. That is the highest mark which is almost inexpressible in words." (see source 29 p. 298-299)

One might imagine that imbalance would arise from living in the West where one's focus is on material goals at the same time as wanting to practice the spiritual wisdom of the Orient. Actually, it is precisely the opposite. Materialism in itself holds no satisfaction, and a person who seeks spiritual nourishment also has need of the physical reality. Babuji used the bird as an image of the right balance: One wing represents the spiritual aspect, the other the physical aspect; the bird needs both wings to be able to fly. And the Master is like the tail which enables the bird to keep on the right course.

One day on a later trip to India, when I was in a scooter-rickshaw on a main road in Chennai, jammed in amongst the Indian rush hour traffic and rather impatient to get back to the ashram, I suddenly saw the whole scenario as an image of this spiritual path: There is room for everyone, regardless of whether they are walking, riding a bicycle, being transported in a dilapidated vehicle or a Rolls Royce.

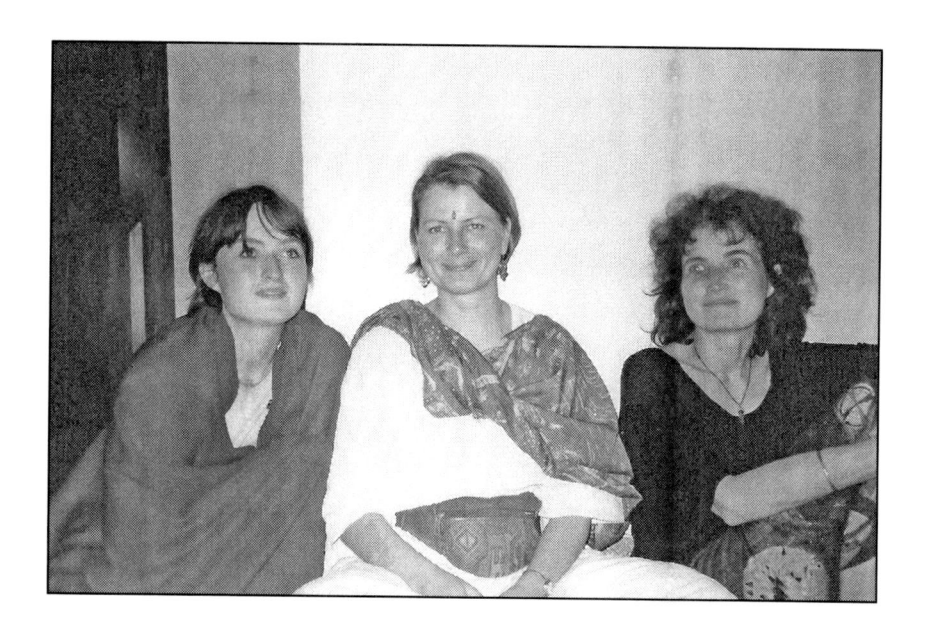

The author with two meditation friends in front of Chariji's home in Madras. Photo: Unknown person who was present, 1997

All the time, people are joining the group and others are leaving it. The biggest and fanciest car is not necessarily the quickest way forward, because it has to adapt itself to the traffic and is often too big and clumsy to be able to choose the shortcuts. When the vehicles are stuck in the traffic jam, the pedestrians can slip elegantly between them and carry on regardless. The unpredictable movements of the traffic demand that everyone pays constant attention. The fumes from one's own and the other vehicles cause physical discomfort as well as an unpleasant mist and fog which prevents the road users from breathing freely and seeing reality clearly. But in spite of these factors, the whole menagerie moves little by little towards the goal. The goal must be clear from the start in order to avoid getting lost in the seething mass. Nothing can be taken for granted in this inferno. There is only one thing to do: identify the goal and surrender to the divine will, trusting that you will get there.

When I was occupied in finishing the work on this book, sitting with my nose buried in the Vedas and the Yoga Sutras, I was suddenly struck by a thought. One of the pieces of information on my palm leaf was that in the future I would study the scriptures of the forefathers. The guru Swamiji had also recommended that I learn about Hinduism etc. At that moment I had to acknowledge that I had unexpectedly followed the directions of both. I had not planned to pass on my experiences in this book on the basis of a desire to make their words come true. But nevertheless, that is what happened.

At the moment I am enjoying the view from the mountainside where I am standing. I did not plan to bind myself to one particular Master, but I am now happy that I did so. The desire to see the world in a larger perspective is always present. It drives me forward on the path to spirituality. The journey is not just about taking part in seminars and trips to India. It is an eternal dialogue with the universe where change is the only predictable thing. As the contact with my mountain guide's heart becomes stronger, I feel more clearly that the seed of happiness is and always has been within myself. I trust that his path will lead to the goal and that I am on the right road. But all these words are just post-rationalisations in an attempt to find explanations which can confirm the choices which my heart has already made. The strong force between the Master and the student does not base itself on logical conviction, but on love. Love is the very stuff of which the path to the goal is made.

Sahaj Marg and SRCM – international

[The following contact information has been updated in 2017.]

The approach to meditation with transmission based on the Sahaj Marg method is today called *Heartfulness*. It means that centres and activities regarding Sahaj Marg meditation in the whole world also carry the name: Heartfulness.

Heartfulness is widespread in all the continents of the earth.

There are both Heartfulness centres and also more local groups where people meet to meditate and receive transmission together.

Information on Heartfulness centres in the whole world can be found on one map – please see this link which can also be accessed via the QR code below:

http://heartspots.heartfulness.org

The link below will take you to your national Heartfulness home page where you can find more information:

http://heartfulness.org

You can read more about Heartfulness via the chapter: "Postscript 2017 – 23 years after the trip" under the subtitle: "Heartfulness".

POSTSCRIPT 2001 – 7 YEARS AFTER THE TRIP

Has the journey in 1994 influence on my life today?

A story gets an extra dimension when you can follow its development through time and reveal whether the conclusions gave lasting results. Therefore, I have chosen to share some of my later experiences to show whether the journey I made back then was instrumental in forming the life I live today. Where am I now in my search for happiness and the truth of life, and how do I now relate to the gurus I met and the messages I was given by the palm leaf astrologer? This is explained in the following ...

How the palm leaf prophecies worked out

In the years that have passed since my visit to the thumb print palm leaf astrologer described here, I have come no closer to a scientific revelation as to how so much information about me could be written on this palm leaf. The experience is still a mystery to me and it has left a deep impression on my mind. As previously mentioned, in particular two of the pieces of information on the leaf affected me deeply when the astrologer read them out in 1994. One was that spirituality always would be the most important thing in my life. That prophecy still holds true and I am convinced that it will continue to do so the rest of my life. The other important information predicted that I would have a son when I was 37 or 38 years old. The following story will show whether this prophecy was fulfilled.

In a previous relationship before my journey to India in 1994 I had not succeeded in getting pregnant, not even with the help of medical science. A benign tumour on my pituitary gland which is hormonally active, caused the value of one of the female hormones to be about 100 times higher than the normal level. I lived with the effects of the tumour for many years before becoming aware that it existed and was the cause of the imbalance. With a condition such as this, which is quite rare, there is little chance of becoming pregnant.

After my return home in 1994 I lived a single life. There was no man in my sights with whom I wanted to start a family. This was the situation when my 37th birthday arrived. Since my return I had not listened to the tape recording from the astrologer. I only remembered that the astrologer had mentioned 37 as the age when I would become a mother. As it did not look as if this prediction would be fulfilled, I was disappointed with the state of things. The only step I could take on my own was to try to correct the hormonal condition in an alternative manner. So I did that, but without any radical results. One day, for some reason or another, I got hold of the tape from the astrologer and listened to it again. Then I was pleasantly surprised to hear that the prediction about my age for possibly giving birth also continued into my 38th year. So in spite of everything there was still a little hope to hold on to.

Time passed and my biological clock was ticking mercilessly. As I was nearing my 38th birthday, there was still no break-through in my situation, neither on a physical level nor with my status as a single woman. For a short time, I had had my eyes on a man. He was a person that I would not immediately have placed in the partner category, but all the same there was a special attraction about him. However, as he turned out to be otherwise engaged, this attraction disappeared and I did nothing to prevent it. I was rather upset about my situation, because it had always been my greatest wish to have children ever since I was a child myself. One day the man in question telephoned and invited me to dinner. He was in town for a short while and it turned out to be a pleasant meeting, so we arranged to meet again the next evening. The next day was to be one of the most important in my life. Out of the blue, he asked me to marry him. I remember thinking: *Perhaps this is the one time in my life when I should be prepared to shut the back door,* which in previous relationships I had always kept open in order to have a chance to escape. In my conception, marriage is a partnership for life. Closing the back door and throwing away the key was naturally a frightening thought, particularly when it comes in such a surprising manner – without any forewarning. But I heard myself say "Yes", however not until after he had repeated his proposal in other words, so I was convinced that he meant it seriously. A few days later I sent a fax to Chariji. He approved the coming marriage and also offered us a spiritual marriage ceremony some months later. After a month or so, I began to feel a little strange. I took a pregnancy test. Although my hormonal state had improved a little, pregnancy was not really a possibility. But to my joyful surprise, the test was positive. At the hospital where I was used to going, the comment was: "It shouldn't really be possible, but you are pregnant, so congratulations". I had become pregnant in the first week that I knew my husband. It was something of a miracle for me that my dreams had been fulfilled in only a few days and precisely at a time when everything was looking black. It was almost as if the child simply wanted to come down to us now and therefore made it happen in spite of physical impediments.

So that is how it came about that at an age of about 37½ I was to give birth to my first child. As my stomach began to grow, various people, independently of one another, would come to me. With a serious look in their eyes, almost all of them said something along these lines: "What a lovely "boy–tummy" you have there. I can see that by the shape, and I'm usually right". Naturally, I was also aware that the little child hiding there probably was a boy.

The months of pregnancy flew by, we were married in India and in Denmark and were also busily occupied in finding a place to live and getting everything in order. We had neither the time nor the opportunity to think or talk about a name for the baby, and both of us preferred to wait until the baby was born. For sometimes you can almost see what a child's name is to be, once it has arrived.

One of the advantages of being the last of my sisters to have a child, was that I could inherit their baby things. The only toy I bought before the birth was a little soft toy – a lamb. You could have the toy with either a red or a blue bow round its neck. I thought the red bow was the nicest. I simply could not make myself choose the blue one, although it probably would have suited the baby best, so I let the saleswoman wrap the one with the red bow.

The time came when the baby was ready to meet us and the world. The night the labour pains started, a thought suddenly struck me. It was: *Signe is also a pretty name*. I had not been thinking about names – I was fully preoccupied with relating to the new and urgent sensations in my body. So my reaction was to think: *What nonsense, it's a boy that's on his way out*, and so I pushed the thought about the name away. Signe was not a name that had previously made an impression on me, but later in the day when the pains became unbearable and I was floating around in a large bath, the thought came to me again: *Signe is a really pretty name*. This time I was even more surprised, because I was only concentrating on the pains when the thought struck me again. All the same, it was strange that the same thought came again almost word for word ... Later that same day, the baby arrived and turned out to be the loveliest girl in the world ... at least that is her mother's opinion. What name other than "Signe" could we give this little new stranger, the name she had told me beforehand? Her strong will and temperament, which I recognised from her time in my womb, matched perfectly the fact that she wanted to choose her own name.

That is how it happened that I gave birth to a child at the time predicted, but the gender was different from what was written on the palm leaf. The toy lamb with the red bow suited our small daughter beautifully. Looking back, it is strange to think that my intuition and inner desire had chosen the "right" colour. Actually, it is great that the predictions were not fulfilled in this respect. Not because the child's gender itself was important – because a boy would have been just as welcome to us – but because it was a great relief for me. If this one piece of information on the leaf did not coincide with reality, then there might be others that did not. Thus the rest of my life was not predetermined. I enjoy having the freedom to live my life unaffected by the words on the leaf.

There is also another factor which makes my future uncertain. The reason is that I have chosen Chariji as my Master and that he is able to intervene in the course of my life. It is a well known fact that if you go to ordinary astrologers, their predictions will no longer be valid when you have bound yourself to this Master.

Would I recommend a palm leaf astrologer?

Everyone must decide something like this for themselves. I think there have both been advantages and disadvantages regarding my experiences in connection with the palm leaf astrologer I visited. It was amazing to experience that something like that could happen. It was also great to see myself and my innermost being illuminated by the description of the astrologer, and it was good to see a light ahead in respect of my great desire to become a mother.

On the conscious level, my daughter's gender made it possible for me to distance myself to the palm leaf's other information about my future. Because she turned out to be a girl and not, as was written, a boy. As this prediction was not correct, I could not completely trust the other information about the future. In some way this was actually a relief. I was satisfied with what life had presented me with – whether it was predicted or not. Therefore, I was surprised one day to discover that the palm leaf prediction continued to influence my condition. Because the information had also lodged itself hidden in my unconscious from where it affected my life. A visit to a kinesiologist, who can decode parts of the unconscious by testing the muscles of the body, 6 months ago showed me that my subconscious mind was still deeply affected by certain of the palm leaf's other prophecies about my future, among others the prediction about my time of death. The kinesiologist made me aware of this other aspect of the palm leaf predictions. That the subconscious mind accepts the words as the truth. In these circumstances, such a "programming" of the subconscious mind can very easily create havoc in one's system. I then made a decision about the prophecy in question and tidied up both the conscious and the subconscious aspect of the matter.

I would not choose to go to an astrologer today. Of course, it is an "easy" time in my life to say this, when I have now had most of my great wishes granted. Perhaps that is why it said that I would come to get the information exactly in 1994 when it meant so much to me.

Latest news on the special palm leaf astrologer

A friend visited the palm leaf astrologer in February 1999. The astrologer was still there, but my friend left without finding out whether there was a palm leaf with his name on it. The reason was that the place had now developed into a rather expensive enterprise. Firstly, Westerners had to pay a basic price which was four times as high as the price for Indians. After that they had now to pay a certain amount for every piece of information on the leaf and as a minimum pay for the four basic pieces of information about parents, spouse, children and time of death. The price for these four basic pieces of information in 1999 was approximately 115 USD plus about 3 USD for the English translation of each answer. The answers to each of the following questions would cost about 30 USD. So if you are considering visiting this special thumb print palm leaf astrologer, the address is still the same, but your purse needs to be a great deal heavier than mine was in 1994 when I paid about 7 USD for all the information.

Newest facts about the gurus I visited in 1994

As mentioned previously, I had many positive experiences and gained many impressions with each of the four gurus I visited. But after I have chosen Chariji as my Master, I no longer have any connection with any of them. However, certain information about the gurus has reached my ears. Below is a short summary of the situation, as far as I know it, with regard to Swamiji, Sai Baba, Amma and Papaji.

Swamiji

Since my return home from the trip in 1994, Swamiji has been to Europe several times. He has also visited Denmark three times – in the summer of 1998, 1999 and 2000 – when he held courses and also gave concerts. I myself did not go to see Swamiji during these visits.

Swamiji's internet address is: http://www.dattapeetham.org

Sai Baba

[Added in 2017: Sai Baba left this physical world on 24 April 2011. There is still activity going on in his main ashram at Puttaparthi. In the years leading up to his death there was a lot of media publicity with allegations that Sai Baba had subjected children to sexual abuse. Personally, I find this hard to believe – and the media can be motivated by other interests in certain cases than seeking the truth. In the wake of these allegations about Sai Baba came all the revelations about the many cases of paedophilia within the Catholic Church. In these and similar cases I think you have feel in your own heart what it is important to listen to. However, it is an indisputable fact that Sai Baba through his work has created schools, hospitals, museums and much more at a purely physical level. His spiritual work for human beings and the world is difficult for us to assess, because we can only see a little of the divine reality.

The internet address is: http://www.srisathyasai.org.in

Amma

[Added in 2017: Amma has become very well-known during the past 17 years. She travels around most of the world and also comes to Europe every year.]

The Indian internet address is: http://www.amritapuri.org
The American internet address with Ammas European tourplan is: http://amma.org/meeting-amma/europe

Papaji

As mentioned, Papaji is no longer among us in his physical form. It is still possible to visit his home and also the house where he used to give satsang-Satsang Bhavan.

The internet address is: http://www.satsangbhavan.net

While Papaji was alive, he recommended an American woman to carry on his work. Her name is Gangaji. I took part in her satsang in

Austria and in Germany in 1993 between my two trips to Papaji. In my experience, she had a fine way of passing on her own insight in the spirit of Papaji.

Her internet address is: http://gangaji.org

My relationship with Sahaj Marg and Chariji today

One of the pieces of information on the palm leaf was that I would return to India again and again. That is correct, for since my journey in 1994 I have visited the country five times to spend time with Chariji. My relationship with Sahaj Marg and Chariji is lifelong and probably even longer. I still carry out the daily practice and always experience that I receive the help I need on my way from this Master. I do not always recognise at first what is happening as being a help. But on looking back it is always so. The best way to describe my present relationship with him is to pass on my impressions and experiences from my latest journey to India which I undertook in the summer of 2001. In every day speech most abhyasis use the word "Master" as synonym for Chariji. I have chosen to do likewise below.

Experiences in Tiruppur, India, 2001

After having my baby I had given up the idea indefinitely of travelling to India to see Chariji again. When a preceptor suggested six months ago that I should go there, I thought the idea was extremely unrealistic. Signe was then only eighteen months and in my opinion too little to come with me. Leaving her seemed impossible to me.

But the idea matured, and the obvious opportunity was to see Master at the birthday seminar at Tiruppur in July 2001. If I arranged the trip efficiently, I could be in Tiruppur during the seminar by just being away from Denmark and Signe for six days.

Spending a lot of money travelling to India and only staying there for five days seemed somewhat extravagant to me, particularly as the money had to be borrowed. And if on top of that Master would be coming to the international seminar in Denmark in August – only almost a week after – it seemed even more foolish. But luckily where the attraction of Master is involved, the sensible thing to do is not always what seems the most pressing. My husband supported the idea of the trip. He would take his holiday and look after Signe at the same time. I knew that she would be happy and safe with her father in my absence. So the journey was within the bounds of possibility. If Master decided to come to Denmark in August, I decided just to be pleased that I would then be able to spend another seminar with him.

Fortunately, I went on this trip which in several ways became a turning point in my spiritual practice. Time has no meaning when you are with Master. This, my shortest trip to India, may have been the most fruitful.

With this long introduction I wanted to give an example of the resistance one can have in connection with translating the idea of a journey to Master into action. At the same time I would urge anyone – who might have this idea – to realise it. Being with Master moves everything into a different dimension. When, after spending one day in Chennai and four days in Tiruppur, I was due to return home again, I had no sensation of having been in India for five days, a week or a month – time is a relative concept, especially when one is close to him.

☙

Compared with Chennai, Tiruppur in Southern India is a small town. Perhaps that is why I imagined before my departure that Master's birthday seminar would be a small one. When I arrived, it turned out that they had made room for 12,000 people and that in actual fact about 17,000 participants came. I was surprised – but not disappointed. This feeling of being unaffected in my innermost self, regardless of what was going on in the outer world, was the inner state in which I found myself throughout the whole seminar. This gift from Master began when the plane from Denmark took off, and lasted until I landed here again. I felt like a little drop of oil in the sea which floated on the surface all the time, regardless of the movements of the water.

Before leaving I had arranged to be picked up in Chennai and driven to Manapakkam – the ashram near Chennai – where I stayed the first night. The next day the driver took me to the airport again from where I continued to Coimbatore. There I was met by Tiruppur abhyasis, because I had informed them in advance of my arrival. We were six abhyasis who shared a taxi to the ashram. In India it is quite normal to have six passengers and one driver in an ordinary taxi. A preceptor among the passengers gave a sitting in the car on the way. In Tiruppur, there were about ten large tents for sleeping which were made of interwoven palm leaves. Fortunately, I caught sight of some Danes in the tent where I wanted to be, because it was close to everything. Later I realised that I had found the best place of all with regard to Danes and western abhyasis that I knew. From the next day, a wedding hall had been rented where the westerners could stay during the seminar. Although it was only a few hundred meters down the road, I preferred to stay in the ashram in the middle of everything.

It is very easy to settle into a seminar if you have travelled in India before. In my luggage I had a mattress to lie on and a mosquito net to build a cosy nest. So I did not need to go looking for the mattress rental place or to stand in several queues. The mosquito net is important, because even though there might not be that many mosquitoes, the space under the transparent mosquito net seems nice and private when you are sleeping alongside men and women, westerners and Indians in the sleeping tent. Earplugs in the sleeping tent are also a "must" for a good night's sleep.

In Tiruppur they had been preparing this seminar for the past six months. Bushes had been cleared away to make room for all the tents. The meditation tent was a large, three-winged, beautifully decorated palm leaf building. If we had had a lot of rain during the seminar, we would probably have been sleeping and meditating in puddles. But luckily all the tents stayed dry during the whole seminar and the weather was on our side. Now and again there was a gentle wind which scattered the light, red road dust everywhere. Every evening you had to remove a layer of dust from your mattress. I soon learnt to put my sheet and the other clothes back in my suitcase when they were not in use. My nose was almost constantly full of red grit. But even this could not in any way affect the exhilaration I felt inside.

The whole seminar was very well-run and well-arranged. Although there were 17,000 participants, the whole thing ran smoothly like one big organism where everything was coordinated, in spite of seeming quite casual. I only noticed the crush in the morning when the queues in front of the bathrooms lasted for hours. Fortunately, the toilet queues were short, and they are, after all, the most important. I enjoyed the scenery in the morning in this crowded women's room where bathing and dressing were carried out in one great confusion. Also the familiar sound of the women's bracelets jingling against each other and the tinkling of the chains around their ankles were music to my ears. It was lucky for me that the customs of the Indians were so predictable. By doing the opposite of them and going to the bathrooms after the evening sitting when the others went to eat, I could enjoy my bath without having to wait. Also the air had become so cool that you could miss out on the morning bath. Moreover, only one bath a day was permitted. There had been a shortage of water in all of Southern India for the past six months, and during the seminar they had to spend a lot of money buying thousands of litres of water every day. There were

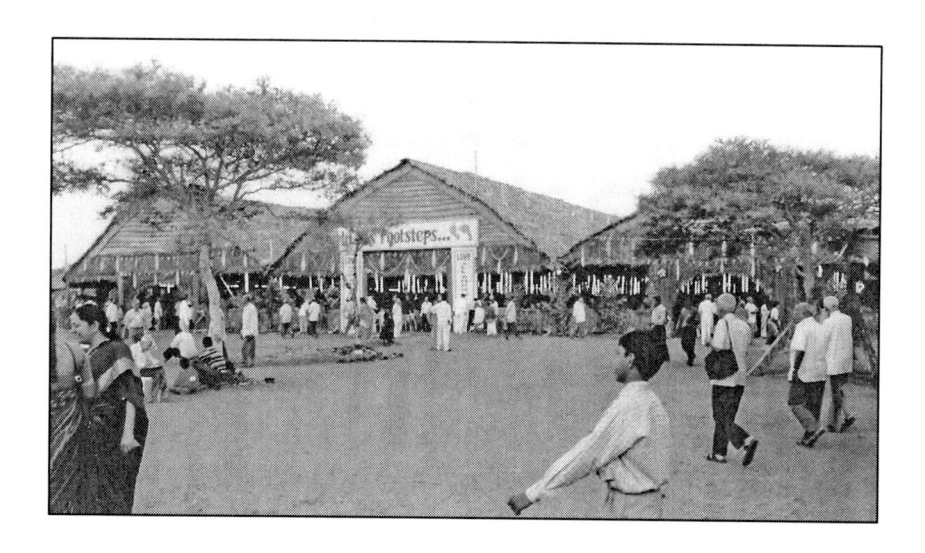

*The three-winged meditation hall in Tiruppur which was
built of palm leaves. Photo: Lisbeth Ejlertsen, 2001*

many food queues and it does not take long in India when they serve the food up on your plate. Water was served at many tables around the ashram and there was a special canteen with other dishes for sale and a café selling ice cream, soft drinks, coffee, snacks etc.

One of my goals on leaving home had been to get more out of my daily practice and to have a closer contact with Master in my heart. After the birth of my daughter I was not satisfied with my own efforts when I was meditating or cleaning. I felt that I was not focussed enough. As at every seminar, it worked out that I got what I was looking for. This time the directions I wanted came to me in the following way:

The first or second day of the seminar I was having lunch with a Danish abhyasi and an Australian man. This Australian suddenly starting talking about his practice, his progress as an abhyasi and his goals with Sahaj Marg. I have seldom met such a goal-oriented abhyasi. His whole day was pervaded by his desire to strengthen his contact with Master. He read Master's books both morning and evening in order to get into the right mood for saying the prayer with the strongest possible impact. When he wanted to smoke a cigarette and could see the cigarette in his mind's eye, he replaced the cigarette image with an image of Master at the same time as intensifying his longing – his "craving" – for what was a cigarette before, but was now Master. In this way he used many every day situations to establish and extend his longing for Master. He had previously been meditating in the system for about five or six years without feeling that he had progressed. So he had stopped for six months and when he then resumed the practice, the impact was completely different. His idea was that it was necessary to clean efficiently first in order to meditate properly. His cleaning method today was to imagine that he was Master and that it was Master, and not himself, who was doing the cleaning. This was only possible, he said, because he had built up a trust in Master that he would be with him at all times. As it was Master doing the cleaning, the man did not have to take responsibility for doing the cleaning "well enough". This gave him the relief he needed. When he was cleaning, he examined his heart region first to see how everything was. After that he focused first on cleaning the heaviest things away and then on things that were more subtle, and so on until most of the subtle dirt had gone. Moreover, the Australian was of the opinion that abhyasis in general did not test Master enough. Because only by putting Chariji to the test and experiencing positive results could one build up one's trust in him, and faith is the foundation for one's further practice.

I could write many pages about this Australian's accounts of his practice and his results. When I tried out his directions at the first given opportunity, I experienced a great difference and a feeling that the cleaning *was* more effective. We carried on our talks during the rest of the seminar and I believe we both found inspiration in that. For it is often the case that people meet each other, because they each have something to give the other. He was in the process of getting a divorce from his abhyasi wife. I questioned discreetly whether this was the right solution to his situation.

Besides a new situation with my own practice I brought a gift home with me to do with Constant Remembrance. Although I knew about this element in the Sahaj Marg method beforehand and even though I had tried it to the best of my ability many times, my understanding of Constant Remembrance had still not taken root completely. For on this trip I became aware on a deeper level why it is so important to be in Constant Remembrance and that it has really nothing to do with Master as the person you see at first glance. Because when you imagine that you *are* him, it happens that you connect simultaneously to his inner state and thus to the eternal source with which he is both connected and at one. By imagining *being* him, you yourself become *connected to this source.*

An idea for an image came to me which I have described below. It illustrates both the Master's capacities and at the same time his ability to help his students. The image contains the following elements from the spiritual practice in the Sahaj Marg method:

- *cleaning* – the exercise we ourselves can use to cleanse our minds.
- *transmission* – the special help we can receive from the Master – "the instrument" he used to remove the effect of old impressions (samskaras) from our inner selves.
- *Constant Remembrance* – the fact that we, through our thoughts and hearts, can connect to the Master when we consciously choose to do so. In this way we come into contact with highest vibration to which he is connected.

In order to paint the picture with which I will illustrate the Master's resources and capacity, the following very rough and simplified comparisons are necessary for the divine source, the Master as well as us ordinary people:

- **The divine source and vibration** – are compared below with a *power station* producing all the electricity for the whole world.
- **The Master** – is identified by being a combination of the following three elements:

  * the *transformer station* that converts voltage from the power station level to the lower level which can be used by everyone in our homes

  * *the electricity grid* i.e. *the supply network* that carries the electricity from the transformer station out to everyone's homes and thus to our electric outlets

  * *the Master lamp*, a large electric lamp equipped with a fine and clear electric light bulb with a powerful light. It is connected to the electricity supply network and can be seen by everyone in the world.

  It is the combination of these three elements which together illustrate the role and capacity of the Master. By being the transformer station he is connected both to the divine source, the power station, and he also converts this strong energy to a level which can be endured by people. Furthermore, by also being the supply network, he passes the energy on in the reduced version which people can endure to use. Last but not least he shows his capacity by the light in the Master lamp which he also is. The strong level of light from the Master lamp fulfils, among other things, the purpose of attracting people's attention and making us want to shine in the same way.

- **The people / the students** – are compared in the following to *battery-powered lamps*. They also have electric light bulbs, but they do not shine as brightly as the Master lamp. Partly because the batteries do not have such a strong capacity as the network supplies, and partly because the light bulbs in the battery powered lamps are dirty. Each battery lamp has only one battery available throughout its whole lifetime. Thus there is a limit to how much light they each can give and how long they can shine.

Although none of the above comparisons can stand a deeper analysis, the image may be of use all the same ... With this in mind, the image of the Master's work and the usefulness of transmission, Constant Remembrance and cleaning can be illustrated as follows:

The Master radiates a bright light via his Master lamp. Its light bulb is clean, therefore it can shine with great effect. The Master lamp shines at full strength always and all of the time. This is possible, because the Master lamp is connected to the electricity supply net which via the transformer station is connected to the power station which is the divine source. The energy there is the highest and it is available all the time.

In the people's battery lamps the light only comes from the one battery which each person has at his/her disposal during this life. These battery lamps only give a limited level of light and they have to economise on the battery so it doesn't get used up too quickly. Furthermore, the light bulbs in these battery lamps are dirty both inside and out. Some people don't know this – others don't think so much about it and they don't have any effective means for removing the dirt. With their lower light capacity they can only see a limited section of what exists around them. Most battery lamps do not realise this either. They think they have seen the whole world and everything in it.

The battery lamps live among each other. They think their light is lovely and good. Only a few know anything about the fact that there exists a lamp which shines brighter than themselves. People don't realise this until the day when they catch sight of the Master lamp.

When people meet the Master, most of them experience a special field around him – a unique and powerful light. It feels light, warm and good to sit near the Master lamp, because it constantly radiates this bright and special light. Everything becomes clearer and more comprehensible when seen in the light of this quite special powerful lamp.

Even though it feels good in every way to sit close to the Master lamp, it does not make the students" own battery lamps able to shine like the Master lamp. To attain this the battery lamps have to go through various phases: firstly they need a cable to connect to the electricity supply network, and secondly they have to choose to connect to the network via a power outlet. In fact the battery lamps already have a cable within themselves, they just don't know it. It is hidden inside their hearts.

*It is the Master's wish that everyone and everything on earth is completely illuminated. He knows that this can only happen when all the battery lamps in the whole world shine at their brightest level. The Master is happy when battery lamps discover that there exists a lamp which shines brighter than themselves. For then he has the opportunity to tell them that they themselves may come to shine as brightly if they so wish. But they have to choose to reach out for it themselves. If they wish to be able to shine at the level of the Master, the first step is to activate their cable. The Master helps them with this too. During the first **transmission**, the Master shows the students that they already have this cable in their hearts and he rolls it out for them.*

*In spite of the fact that the cable is available to the battery lamps, it is still not enough to shine powerfully. Not until the students put the cable into the power outlet – via **Constant Remembrance** – will their own lamp start to shine at a level similar to that of the Master. Because then they are connecting to the electricity supply network at the same time as the Master, and via this to the transformer station which is also a part of the Master's capacity, and through this to the power station which is the divine source. If they should forget to think about the Master, then at the same time they remove their plug from the power outlet again. As they are no longer connected to the supply network and, consequently, not to the transformer station, neither are they connected to the power station. Then they only shine via their own battery again at the lower level. It can take a long time before they find out that the light around them is reduced. When they discover this and when they want to shine with a stronger light again, they just have to think of the Master again. In this way they are putting their cable – via Constant Remembrance – into the power outlet once more.*

The battery lamps which have realised the usefulness of putting their cable into the power outlet and thus again getting access to shining all the time, still do not shine as powerfully as the Master lamp. This is because their electric light bulbs are dirty on both sides of the glass. Because it is the Master's wish that all lamps should shine at the brightest strength, he gives instructions as to how the battery lamps can clean the outside of their light bulbs. By means of **the cleaning** *the battery lamps can reach the outside of the glass themselves and keep it clean. The more carefully this cleaning is done, the cleaner the surface of the light bulb becomes and the brighter it shines.*

Many battery lamps do their utmost and even though some manage to get the surface completely clean, there are still no battery lamps that can shine as powerfully as the Master lamp. This is due to the dirt on the inner side of their light bulb to which they do not have access. This dirt stems from the time they were made. Some were made in a workshop with a lot of dirt, others under cleaner conditions. Although some have more dirt than others, they all have a certain amount of dirt on the inside. This dirt can be removed for them by the Master lamp. This work is also carried out by the Master lamp via **transmission**. *It is impossible to describe how the Master is able to activate and use this special transmission for this purpose. Each battery lamp must decide for itself whether it wishes to test this deep cleansing and see whether it gives any noticeable effect. By observing the other battery lamps that often take this deeper cleansing, the newly arrived battery lamps can perhaps get an idea of whether the cleansing has an effect. They can see whether the lamps which have often been cleaned have attained a fine and powerful light. No matter what, they will not know the effect of cleansing for sure until the day they it try it themselves and feel its effect.*

The battery lamps which clean their light bulbs both on the outside by their own efforts and on the inside by transmission from the Master lamp and that keep their cable constantly in the power outlet via Constant Remembrance, still do not get to shine with the same intensity as the Master lamp. They do not have the same capacity. Because when it comes down to it, they still cannot connect their cable directly to the power station, the voltage is much too high for that. They need the electricity supply network for contact and for the protection which the transformer gives them. If they try to connect directly to the power station, it will all go wrong – their light bulbs will burst and they will not be able to shine any more in this life. For the power station sends out electricity at a very high voltage of at least 1,000 volts and the battery lamps and their cables can, for example in Denmark, only stand 220 volts. Therefore they need help from the transformer station that reduces the voltage level from 1,000 volts to 220 volts, and they also need the electricity supply network that distributes the power to the power outlets in the homes of the battery lamps where they can make use of the electrical energy in peace and with no risk.

It is only because the Master is of a special calibre that he can stand the direct contact with the power station. He has developed the ability to be the transformer and the electricity supply network as well as the Master lamp in one and the same person. He can stand the direct connection to the power station – the most powerful energy – and he transforms the vibration from the highest level to a level which people can stand. Furthermore, he gives help via transmission. By means of this, each individual receives exactly the right amount at the right level of vibration from the highest source which the person in question has the capacity to receive.

Some battery lamps may think: if I just make do with receiving transmission now and again, then my light level will probably be maintained at a good level without my having to do anything else ... But that's not the way it is. Dirt will keep collecting on the outside of its light bulb and if it is not removed daily, its light level will be significantly reduced. In addition, each battery lamp will be left to rely on its own battery and its low capacity again if it does not keep its plug in the power outlet. Therefore: without cleaning, Constant Remembrance and transmission from the Master lamp no battery lamp will radiate light at its optimal level. In this world there is no particular requirement for anyone to shine at any particular level. It is completely up to each individual battery lamp whether or not it wishes *to shine more powerfully and attain, among other things, clarity to find the right path and to walk it more steadily ...*

ಌ

Chariji explains again and again that we should not lose ourselves in his outer form. If we wish to become like him, we must follow his instructions and do what he does. When we achieve being in Constant Remembrance and thus in direct contact with the divine essence, the Master continues to give more help as we carry on our way. He keeps an eye on us, reaches out his hand and lifts us up from the potholes. We need this so as not to get lost in blind alleys on the path of spiritual development – mistakes which can create barriers for our further development.

My experience during the seminar was that when I was sitting in the meditation tent with my eyes closed, I could feel a close connection with Master. When I opened my eyes and looked at Him in his physical form, this sense of togetherness disappeared. As my focus shifted from the inner to the outer level, there was immediately so much distraction that I forgot to hold on to the inner connection at the same time. The art of being present on both levels requires practice. I still have a lot to learn ...

ಌ

During the seminar, Master gave two speeches and several new books were published. I will mention two of them here. One was a collection of letters, articles and the like from Lalaji which had not previously been published as a whole. Master held one of his two speeches in connection with the release of this book from the first Master of the system.

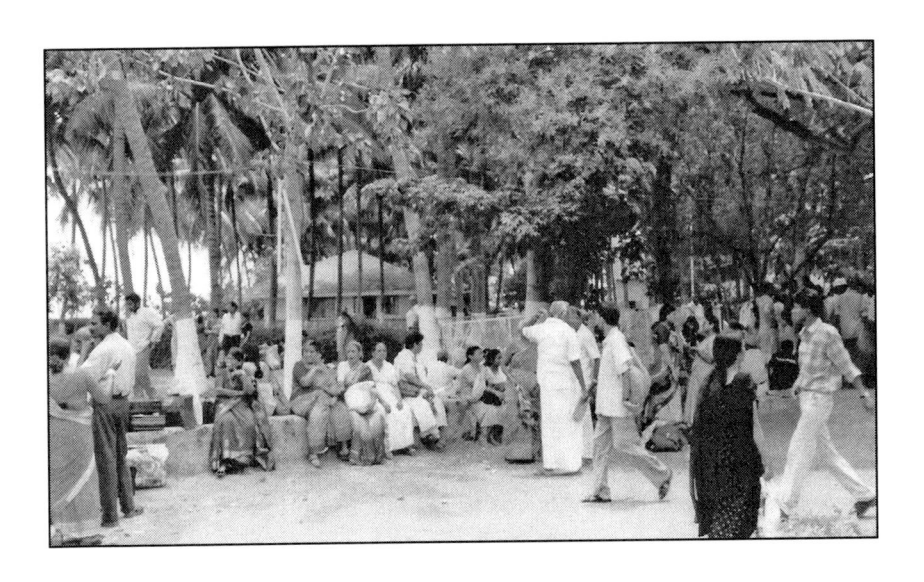

Chariji's house in the background and abhyasis in front as near as they could get to the house. Photo: Lisbeth Ejlertsen, 2001

The book *The Complete Works of Ram Chandra (Lalaji Maharaj)*

Thanks to the kindness of Lalaji's grandchildren, the mission had received the texts and the copyrights for Lalaji's books and writings which previously only existed in Indian languages. This is, therefore, the first time that the material is published in English. In his speech, Master appealed to the readers to just enjoy the book and treat it as an experience. It is an expression from another time, and the methods which Lalaji used belong to that time and not to ours. Therefore, Chariji did not want us to begin to try out the methods which Lalaji refers to. He also warned against making a myth out of Lalaji by mistakenly assuming that because Lalaji was the first guru in the system, he also was the best. Instead Chariji stressed that the Sahaj Marg system, as it is today, is the optimum practice which Babuji established according to Lalaji's direction, even though it happened after Lalaji had left his physical body.

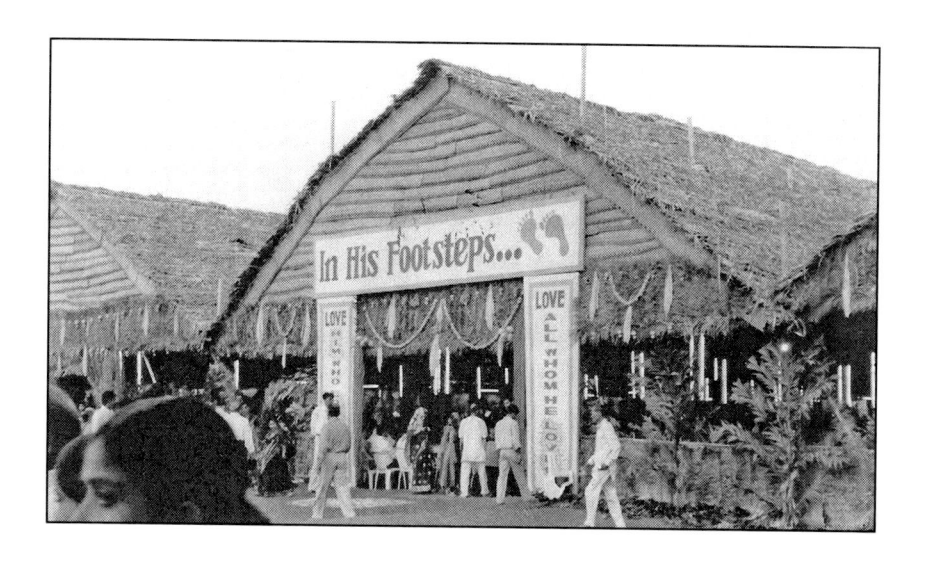

The middle building of the meditation hall with the title of the seminary written above the entrance. Photo: Lisbeth Ejlertsen, 2001

The book *Heart to Heart, Volume IV of Parthasarathi Rajagopalachari (Chariji)*

It was Santosh Khanjee – one of the senior abhyasis from the US – who spoke on the publication of this book. In short, his speech was an appeal to all present to go back to our local centres and there read out Master's predictions from 1990. I have not been able to find a chapter in the book about the predictions from 1990, but there is a chapter on Guru Purnima Day which I think is what he was referring to. It takes up half a page and goes as follows below. But first a few facts on what "Guru Purnima dag" is: The day with this name occurs every year in June-July, but not on exactly the same date. The date is decided by Purnima, the day of the full moon in the Hindu Shanka calendar called the Ashadas month. It falls in June-July. From ancient times this is the day when students express their devotion and gratitude to their guru. The guru's gesture to the students on this day is to bring them a big step further on their path of spiritual development. This is what Chariji had written in the new book about this special day.

Guru Purnima Day, Augerans, France, 8 July, 1990

"*Today, in India, it is the "Guru Purnima" day. It's the day of the full moon, and dedicated to the Guru, supposed to be a very important day in the spiritual life of an abhyasi. Abhyasis who can be with their Master on such a day are considered to be very blessed.*

I take this opportunity of conveying to you my Master's blessings on this very auspicious day. At the same time, I have to charge you all with the responsibility of making use of your spiritual opportunities in the right way and not go about Sahaj Marg in a merely mechanical way. But please, pay attention to your inner character changes that are very necessary, and without which real progress cannot come.

May Master bless you". (see source 32 p. 181)

Master held his second speech on the day of the birthday itself. It seemed as if the idea for it arose spontaneously. When the sitting was over, there were to be music events which Master stayed to listen to. But before the music got started, many Indians got up and tried to make their way out among the other abhyasis who were sitting down. An attempt was made from the microphone to get them to sit down, but without success. Then Master gave a sign that he wanted to speak. That got most of them to sit down again and listen to the scolding which was also part of the speech. In broad outline, Master appealed to everyone to take good care of their bodies. This would aid us in fulfilling our purpose of being here on earth and not, therefore, add further complications to our lives. In general, he asked us to live in moderation in *every* way. As far as the amount of food we consume is concerned, Chariji mentioned that we could all make do with eating 20% of what we normally eat. With regard to our consumption of the world's resources in the form of water, electricity and other material things, he also asked us to reduce our use of these as much as possible.

At the same time I also felt that the speech was an indirect reference to the behaviour of the abhyasis in relation to Chariji's presence. During the whole seminar he stayed in his house which was screened off, and he only came out for the sittings. The reason for this was obvious. It was not a free choice on the part of Chariji, it was a necessary step because of the behaviour of many of the abhyasis. At the times when Chariji was leaving his house to go to the meditation tent and give sittings, the abhyasis gathered together and formed a corridor for him from the house to the meditation hall. It could be a really fine gesture, but this human chain developed every time into something quite out of control. When Master approached everyone wanted to get close to him and touch him. Sometimes it almost seemed as if Master was being crushed. So it was understandable that the screen around his house was placed so that it kept most of us at least 30 meters away. In comparison it is good that Chariji can move around freely in the ashram in Denmark and other places in the world where people do not have the mistaken and antiquated idea that physical contact with the Master is essential for one's spiritual progress.

"In his Footsteps" had been chosen as the title of this birthday seminar. On the birthday itself, communal singing was played when Master entered the meditation tent. We had been asked in advance to clap in time. On the tape there was a choir singing lyrics of which I only remember fragments. As far as I remember, the chorus was as follows:

"There will be footsteps walking with me,
footsteps I cannot see,
everywhere I go,
every step I take,
there will be footsteps walking with me."

At first I felt resistance to this performance, but the tune was lively and catchy, so I wanted to hum along anyway. What I then experienced was that the words went to my heart and tears came to my eyes, because it became very clear at once that Master is with us everywhere we go, often without us noticing.

Together with the song they revealed a new scenery construction which was a copy of Master's patio outside his private house in Chennai, Gayatri. In the same way that Master himself had made a copy of Babuji's veranda in the meditation hall at Manapakkam, the ashram in Chennai, the Tiruppur abhyasis wanted with this gesture to do everything they could for Master to feel at home and comfortable here with them. In his speech he praised them warmly for organising all of this fine and efficient seminar.

To conclude my experiences from Tiruppur I would like to mention my reunion with one of my fellow passengers in the taxi from the airport to the seminar. He was a fairly new abhyasi from another Indian centre – a young man in his mid-twenties. On the second day I met him again while he was standing in the canteen sharing out water to the guests who were buying food. His whole face shone like the sun and he told me that he had practically been working as a volunteer ever since he arrived. He had hardly had any sleep and he had not had time to go to the group sittings. With complete conviction he told me that you get everything you need and can wish for when you work during a seminar. I was deeply touched by his attitude and the visible proof of his answer. In this way he, as a more experienced abhyasi, was a fine symbol of the diligent and gentle spirit which also reigned among the hosts and many other participants at this seminar.

My search for happiness and the truth in life

Here, seven years after my journey to India in 1994, I am living a life much like many other people, with a husband and child, a house and home and also problems. Association with Chariji does not protect you from conflicts and frustrations, because our capaciousness grows when the safe boundaries to which we are accustomed are overstepped.

But the problems do not get to become as massive and long-lasting as before. They are minimised and often disappear when I become aware and let go of my expectations. On the inner level, I choose today to regard all events from the perspective of what these episodes reveal about me and how I can use this information to change my character and liberate myself from old bad habits. The less flotsam and jetsam I carry around, the easier it is to maintain a peaceful inner being.

This attitude to life has made my life something quite special. Other people's doings, which I sometimes find inappropriate and would have reacted to before, now become "gifts" instead of "bad experiences". I willingly admit that it is often the case that I do not experience everything as a "gift" at first. But I am very eager to look for the gift in everything and I keep on searching until I finally find the gift. The value of these gifts is to show me what lies hidden in my personality which needs to be worked on. The desire for development supported by an ever stronger connection to my Master has become the central aspect of my life, while everything else and all other relationships move around this and contribute to my development towards him.

Metaphorically, the spiritual attitude to life can be described as follows: Once you have discovered that films are also available in colour, the black and white versions no longer have any attraction. Similarly, when the spiritual perspective makes life's opportunities unfold like a never-ending colour palette, it is no longer interesting to just regard life on the basis of a perspective in black and white consisting of the limited "materialistic" and apparently "realistic" framework. It is much more interesting to paint your life in colour by exploring new ideas and experiencing what happens when antiquated boundaries are overstepped.

If anyone were to ask me today whether I am a happy person, I can only answer: "Yes!" For a long time I have tended to compare being happy with a feeling of thriving and well-being. Today I would say that happiness is having a Master, because he is always there, regardless of how I feel and what life has to offer me. At the moment my well-being is at a peak, because life is full of so many opportunities which I look forward to exploring. But if anyone had read my well-being barometer a year ago, the mark would have been somewhat lower. Then I was undergoing a tough process of acknowledging and surmounting some deep-lying and grim bad habits.

Any situation in which you find yourself, can be changed completely the moment you yourself change your perspective on what is happening. That is why happiness is having a Master who is always with you and leading you unscathed through even the most difficult moments. What you experience on this path towards realisation is not always so pleasant. The means to carry on and move things forward is honesty in the form of the desire to see what *is* as well as the will to want to overcome your limitations and carry on towards the goal.

The Indian culture has given me the structure for my understanding of the contexts of life, but most of all India is the country which has given me the key to the meaning of life – it is there my Master was born and still lives. Following Chariji's directions constantly opens up for a deeper contact with reality – the greater my effort, the more I get from him in return. Today happiness for me is being with Chariji in my heart and experiencing the truth in life which is gradually revealed, because I am searching for it.

My goals now and in the future

It cannot be said more simply than Chariji has done with these words in source 34, page 22:

"We must be very careful that we don't ask our Master for gifts of power, gifts of happiness, but we ask Him for Himself. Only Love can make this possible."

POSTSCRIPT 2017 – 23 YEARS AFTER THE TRIP

Chariji remained my Master

22 years have now passed since my experiences on my journey to India in 1994. Throughout this long period I kept in contact with Master Chariji. It is, therefore, a matter of importance for me to clarify that my meeting with Chariji was not just a short flirt. My relationship with him only became stronger and more intense in the course of the past 22 years. An abundance of special experiences have each in their own way been contributing factors to the great joy and love in which I constantly evolved and intensified my relationship with Chariji. I visited this Master as often as I have found possible. It amounted to more than 20 journeys to India throughout the years as well as participation in numerous seminars in Europe and also Denmark where he was a regular visitor. My heart is filled with deep gratitude for the support and help Chariji has given me throughout all these years, as he was the living Master for our association and the Sahaj Marg system of meditation.

In December 2014 Chariji left his physical body at an age of 87 years (1927-2014). His health had weakened over a long period of time. I am sure that it was a relief for him to be released from all the limitations that life on earth places on a physical body. I feel very strongly that Chariji is still around me in spirit, around everyone in our association and all other people on earth. For when your aim is to support the whole of humanity in lifting the energy and attaining the highest spiritual level, the work still goes on, even in the spiritual dimension of which he is now a part.

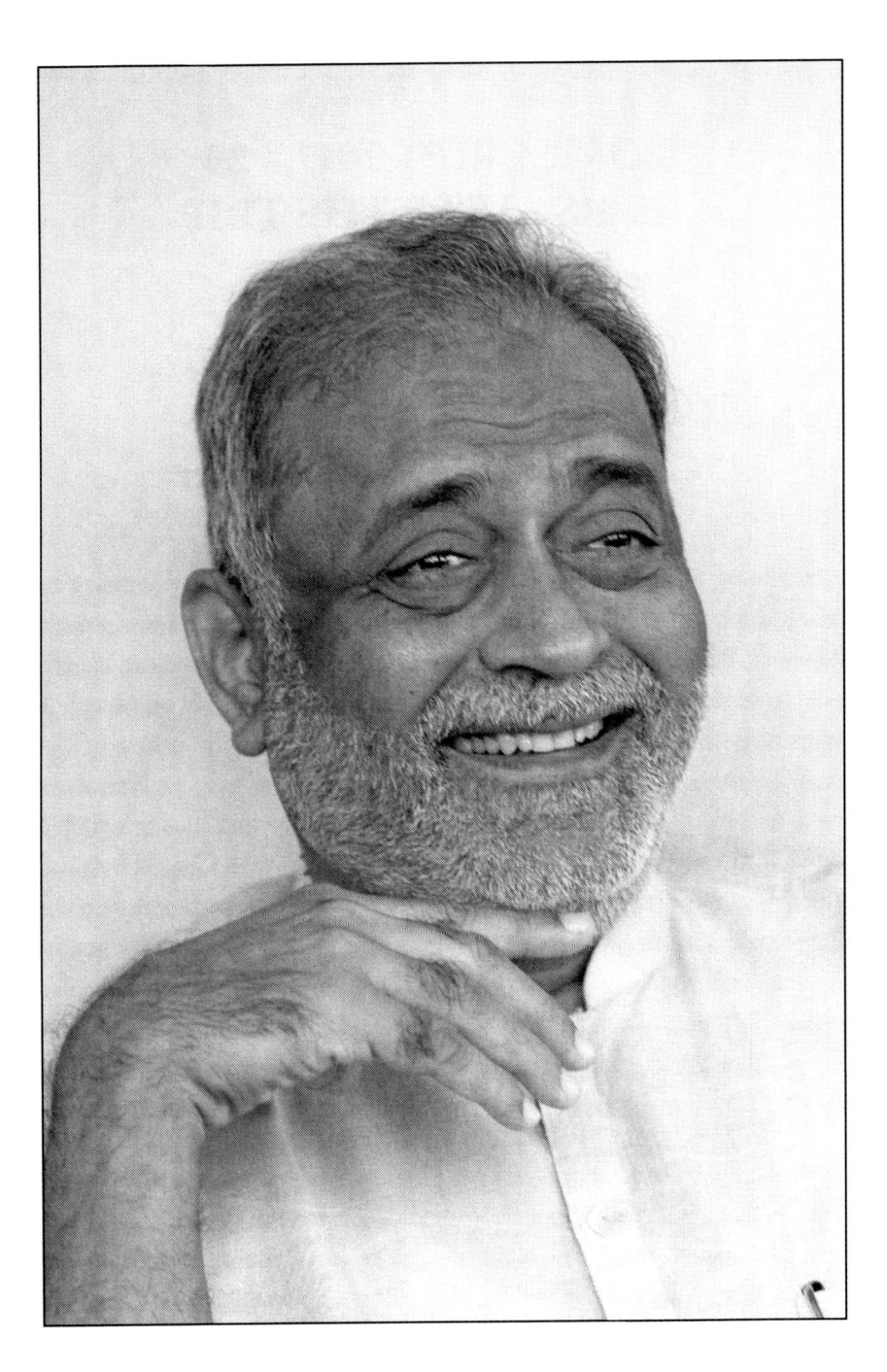

Daaji. See source IX

Chariji's successor: Kamlesh D. Patel – Daaji

For several years Chariji had been preparing the person who was to take on the task after him and thus continue the line of Masters in this association. His successor, the current living Master for SRCM, is Kamlesh Desabhai Patel, born in 1956. He is of Indian origin, studied in the US, and after completing his training as a pharmacist he continued his career in the US and lived there for many years. He is married with two sons who today are adults. These days, he is a global citizen, with his base in India.

I remember vividly the day that Kamlesh was appointed. I had not logged on to the Internet that day before going to the evening sitting at our centre. I had no idea what was happening. Just before the sitting was about to begin, the preceptor stood up in front of the gathering and told us about the announcement on the Internet, and that Kamlesh was to follow in Chariji's Master-footsteps on the day that he would leave his earthly life.

For many – myself included – this was an overwhelming piece of news. I was happy and relieved to hear that there would be a new Master one day when Chariji was no longer here, but I had not previously experienced having to change my attention and love from one Master to another. Among all the teeming thoughts I immediately felt a deep impact on my heart. This calmed my mind to a certain point. My head was trying hard to sort out who exactly Kamlesh was. I recognised the name and knew that I had heard it mentioned several times, because this man had often accompanied Chariji on his journeys here. But there were always a number of men of Indian appearance among Chariji's travelling companions and I could not connect the name Kamlesh with any of them for sure. A face did in fact pop up, but I chose to brush it aside. For if it did not belong to Kamlesh, I did not want to relate myself to this person. I decided to go home first and find out what Kamlesh actually looked like, before relating to him.

But that's not exactly what happened ... Even though your head makes a decision, your body and mind often go their own way regardless of the plans in your head. During the evening meditation which started just after the message about Kamlesh's new status, the image of that Indian face kept looming up in my mind. And it wasn't only the fact that I kept seeing his face. His whole figure had taken a place in my heart. He was there together with the other Masters in our system: Lalaji, Babuji and Chariji. It was as if all four were in a symbiosis with each other – regardless of the fact that two of them still existed in our physical world, while the other two no longer had an earthly body. I could only interpret this vision, which arrived without any conscious help from my side, to mean that Kamlesh was already firmly established in this group of Masters. Finally, I surrendered to the inner knowledge that this face that I was seeing, in actual fact belonged to Kamlesh. When I got home after the sitting and logged on to the Internet and saw Chariji's nomination of Kamlesh, I was happy to learn that it was Kamlesh that I had seen in my mind's eye. This experience resulted in my heart and mind not giving the least resistance to accepting Kamlesh as the new Master when the time came for Chariji to be moving on in the spirit.

During the time leading up to Chariji's farewell to this world Kamlesh began to assume a much larger and more visible role in our association. He often sat at Chariji's side during the group sittings. It was wonderful to see the love, respect and harmony shining from their joint existence. Via the Internet and in speeches Kamlesh began to advise us as to how we can become more aware of our own practice and that our own efforts are crucially significant for our spiritual development. Right from the start I liked Kamlesh's clean and specific instructions and his encouragement to each of us to wake up to our own responsibility. When you have been practising in the same way for years, it can be useful to be shaken up a little – or a lot – so that your practice and efforts do not become apathetic and routine-like. Although love for Chariji filled my whole heart and my ego wanted to keep him for ever as my Master, nevertheless Kamlesh had made his entry there.

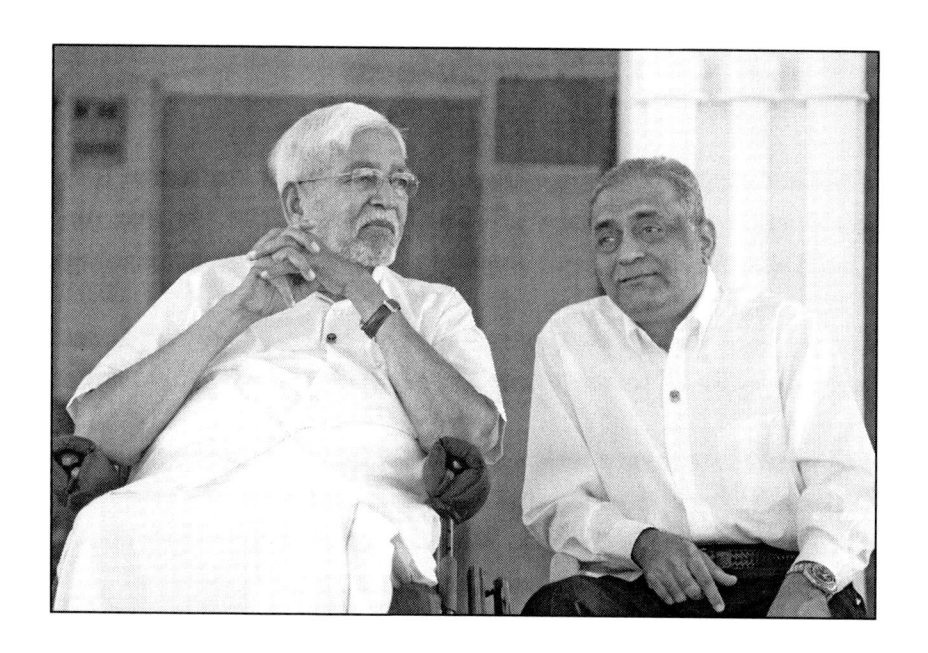

Chariji and Daaji. See source IX

For the rest of the time up to Chariji's farewell they shared the place with Babuji and Lalaji although I had never met the first two Masters in their physical form. Now, a little less than two years after Chariji moved on in the spirit, all four are still in my heart. Therefore, it makes perfect sense to me when the Masters repeatedly affirm that they all four are one.

As with all the previous Masters, Kamlesh does not care to be called "Master". Today he is commonly known as "Daaji", an affectionate name in some parts of Gujarat in India for father's younger brother. The age of the younger uncle is more close to one's own, and therefore it is easier to confide in and seek advice with him. When the Master is seen in that light, it becomes easier for the student to be more receptive to help from the Master.

Heartfulness

The most significant change Daaji has made in our association is the introduction of the concept of Heartfulness in 2014. At that time Chariji was still alive and this new step was taken with his full blessings.

Today Heartfulness is *the* approach to Sahaj Marg, providing an open-hearted way for all seekers to experience what Sahaj Marg has to offer.

The word Heartfulness makes it easier for new people who hear it for the first time to understand that it has something to do with the heart. Then they are already on track. When Heart is connected to fullness it also indicates that there is something special in the heart: a full heart, what the heart is full of or perhaps fullness of the heart ...

There is nothing really new in Heartfulness other than it encourages all of us to participate more actively in sharing Sahaj Marg with the world. As for accessibility, Heartfulness has a lot more to offer, including possibilities provided by modern media.

What Heartfulness offers

Meditation can be started at the age of fifteen and in groups
The age at which seekers can start Sahaj Marg through the Heartfulness approach is now fifteen instead of eighteen, to address the requests from more and more young people to meditate. Also, because of the growing numbers of people who are coming to the practice, most of the meditation sessions are now done in groups – sometimes very large groups of thousands – so as not to limit the number of people who can experience the Master's transmission.

Scientific approach
The Heartfulness approach is very scientific, to resonate with the 21st century, and new seekers are asked to experience meditation first

without transmission, followed by meditation with transmission, so they can experience for themselves the differences.

The means – also two App's
The means by which you can start Sahaj Marg through the Heartfulness approach are more varied using the technology of today: there are two mobile phone applications called "Let's Meditate" and "Heartfulness". The first is so that you can have meditation sessions with a trainer remotely at any time, and the second has audio files of the practice to guide you when you are practising on your own. There are websites and many local social media pages so that you can easily find out what events are happening locally and stay in contact with your local community.

Heartfulness Connect programs
The Heartfulness approach also offers the Heartfulness Connect programs through which workshops are regularly conducted in corporate and government organisations, schools, colleges and universities, neighbourhoods, local communities and villages around the world.

Relaxation exercise
With Heartfulness also comes a new relaxation exercise, which is derived from Patañjali's yoga, but with slight changes as *sankalpa* (a Sanskrit word for subtle suggestion) is used to give each instruction. When we begin, we focus first on the omnipresent energy, especially the energy emanating from Mother Earth. And then we try to imbibe that energy coming upward through our feet, allowing each organ to relax, each muscle to relax, each joint to relax. We proceed from the toes all the way up to the top of the head. And during this process, as one of our trainers is giving the relaxation instructions, they also work on us in a different way by connecting themselves with the Divine Source.

The energy that is flowing upwards from Mother Earth, combined with the connection of the trainer who is conducting the relaxation with the Source, doubly intensifies the relaxation process. A person who has undergone the experiment is touched by both the energy coming from Mother Earth and the energy descending from the Source. They imbibe that impact, and whenever they also conduct such relaxation programmes, they are able to create that immediate impact of relaxation.

As so many people experience stress in the society of today, this relaxation method has been very well received. It only take 5 to 7 minutes and can be done anywhere, anytime, by children as well as adults.

Free of charge
Practising Sahaj Marg through the Heartfulness approach continues to remain free of charge, as is the spiritual tradition. There is no fee to start or to continue.

Heartfulness Institute
Although Sahaj Marg as a practice has always been, and will always be, free of charge, there are many costs associated with the programmes, events and infrastructure currently being offered through Heartfulness. These are organised through the Heartfulness Institute, which now exists in Europe, North America, India, Australia and other countries.

Heartfulness Magazine

The Heartfulness Magazine is an international monthly magazine containing articles about self-development, vitality, relationships, work and living in tune with nature. There are articles about scientific findings, spiritual insights and inspiration from the lives of people who have made a difference to humanity over the ages. For children there are activities and stories that will keep them guessing.

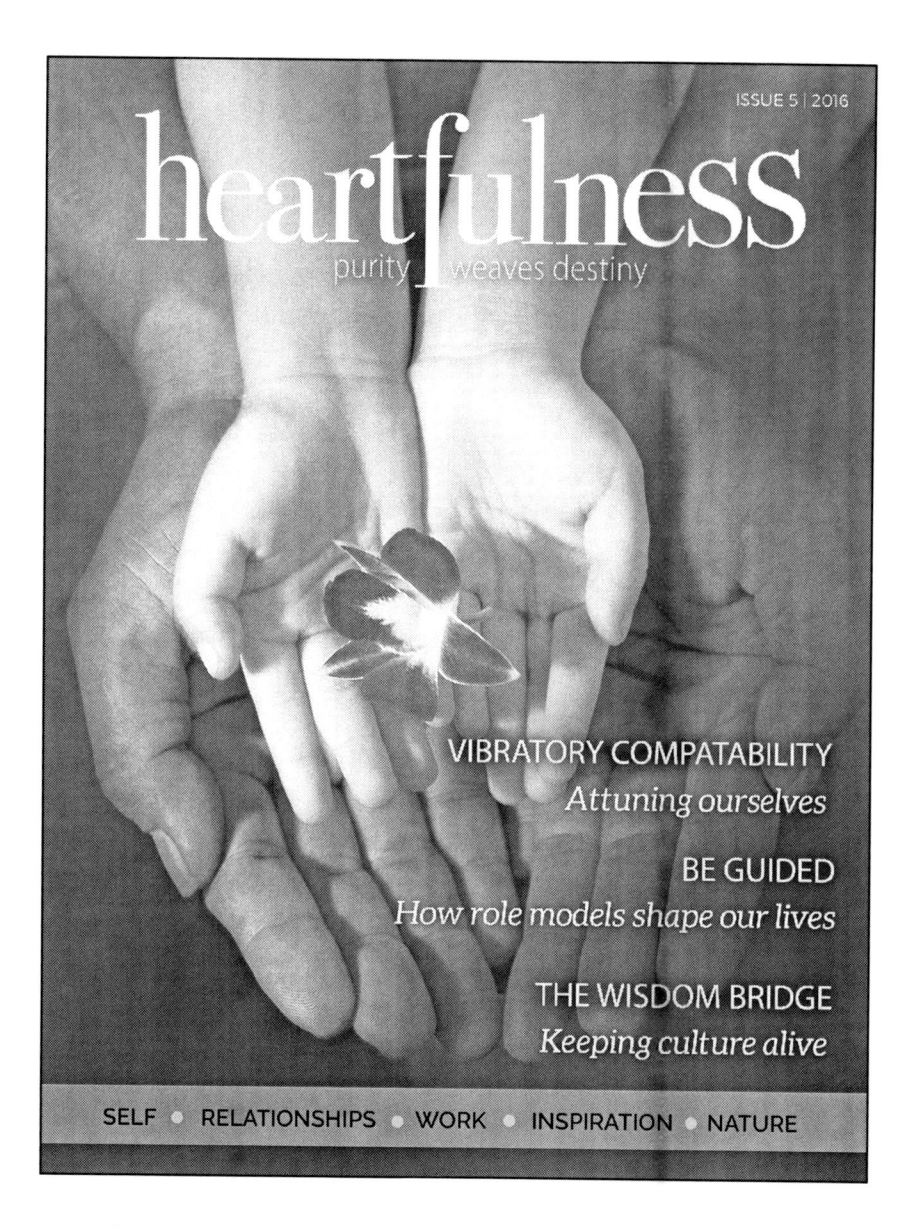

The cover of Heartfulness Magazine issue 5 from 2016. See source IX

The Heartfulness Magazine is available in both digital and print formats. You can subscribe for the e-magazine for free. One of the advantages of the digital version is the possibility to search for a topic across the various issues.

The Heartfulness Magazine is also available in the following languages: French, Chinese, Russian, Portuguese and German.

Heartfulness – towards the future

Sahaj Marg has always been for everyone, and now, through the Heartfulness approach, we are seeing that is has become very accessible for all. As a result, this spiritual path is no longer just the Sahaj Marg method associated with SRCM as an organisation. Heartfulness today has become a movement that is sweeping the world.

With Heartfulness there is room to be exactly the person you are. There are no demands or requirements, only the acceptance and understanding that we are all taking whatever next step on our way we are ready for. According to an old proverb: "Praise not the day before night", it may not be until the day we leave this life that we perhaps can see the path and the meaning for the steps we have taken. We know even less about other people's paths. Each person must follow their own heart. We can only practise listening to and accommodating each other as fellow travellers, following the guidelines charted by the Master to the best of our ability.

Heartfulness logo

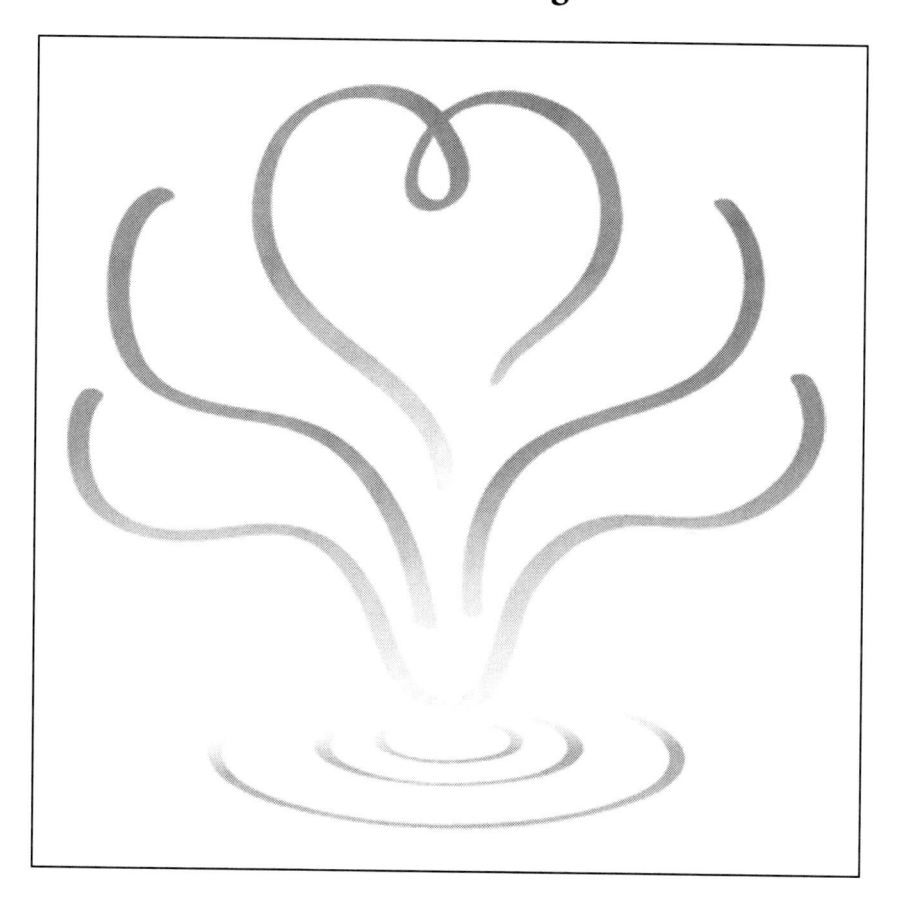

The Heartfulness logo. See source XI

Further information

For further information, please make use of the following services. The various Internet addresses can also be accessed via the QR codes given below each of them.

General information:
For general information and to find out about the practice and explore, please see:

www.heartfulness.org

Find a trainer or centre:
To find a local trainer or centre, please see:

http://heartspots.heartfulness.org

Learn more about Daaji:
To learn more about Daaji, read his articles and listen to his videos, please see:

http://daaji.org

You can also follow Daaji on Facebook, Twitter, Instagram, LinkedIn and Google+.

The two apps:
"Let's Meditate" and "Heartfulness" are available on both Android and Apple phones. Please go to the App Store on your phone and search for those names. The "Heartfulness" app has the subtitle "Heartfulness Institute". You will see the Heartfulness logo in the picture.

You can also download the apps via you PC. Please choose one of following two links which matches the operating system of your phone:

Android:

https://play.google.com/store/apps/details?id=com.htc.heartnew

iOS/Apple:

https://itunes.apple.com/us/app/heartfulness/id1053164680?mt=8

The Heartfulness Magazine:
For the Heartfulness Magazine – please see:

www.heartfulnessmagazine.com

If you want to subscribe for the free e-version of the Heartfulness Magazine – please use:

http://www.heartfulnessmagazine.com/subscribe/

All previous issues of the Magazine can be downloaded from this web site:

http://www.heartfulnessmagazine.com/issues/

New book in autumn 2017: 22 years with the Master

In autumn this year the next volume of the story of my spiritual path will be published. It will be called *The Spiritual Wisdom of India, Volume 2* with the subtitle *22 years with the Master and the Path of the Heart – Heartfulness*.

It is still an unusual step in the West to bind one's heart strings to a Master of Indian origin. This is why I would really like to paint a picture of the gifts and inner happiness such a relationship can bring – to describe that relationship and the path that has unfolded between just an ordinary person from the West like me and a spiritual Master of the highest calibre. At this time when the present book is about to be published in a new edition as well as in English, it would be natural to add a postscript to shed some light on this fact.

At the beginning of this book I referred to one of the usual perceptions many Westerners have of Indian gurus and their followers; that the guru exploits his students who follow their leader blindly like a flock of "silly sheep" without any thought or critical appraisal. As there is no way I can recognise my own relationship with my Master in this perception and as the reality, therefore, is completely different, I would like to break down these prejudices – preferably for all time! At no time have I perceived myself as acting like a "silly sheep" just following an ignorant flock. Every step I have taken towards Chariji has been taken after strict consideration. I have tested his capacity in every direction. Each time I have been amazed by all the experiences that bear witness to the fact that he seemingly works in many dimensions. I would like to share many of the special experiences which have been part of creating the substance of my relationship with Chariji and also with Daaji. Experiences which also show that there is more in heaven and earth than most people imagine.

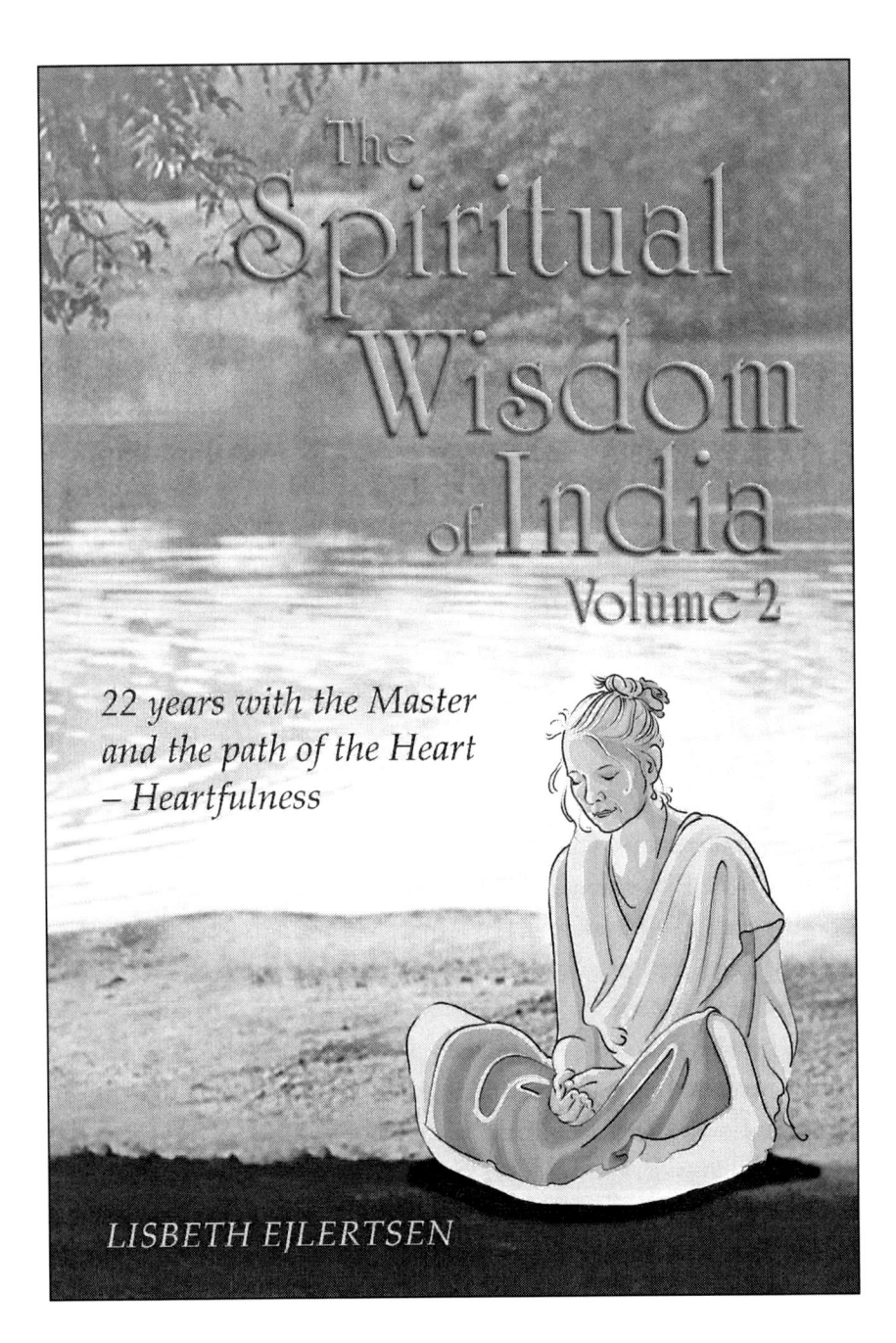

The cover of the next volume of this book:
"The Spiritual Wisdom of India, Volume 2" with the subtitle:
"22 years with the Master and the path of the Heart – Heartfulness"

However, it quickly became clear to me that all these personal experiences could in no way be pressed into a postscript in continuation of this book. Therefore I have chosen to pass them on in a completely new book – a continuation of my spiritual journey and inward search into my heart. In it I would like to take you with me to my physical meetings with the Masters and also to the inner experiences.

The cover photo of this book – originally photographed by Sven Ulsa – shows an old Indian man standing tranquilly looking out across a lake. Although he is looking at the external landscape, you feel that his awareness is equally directed towards the inner depths of his mind. I do not know the old man, but I am very fond of the picture. It symbolises my experiences in India in 1994: a journey out into the word that moved me deeply in my innermost being.

The cover for the new book is shown in the figure. Since 1994 the aim of my journeys to India has been to visit one special Master. Volume 2 is about his work and my experiences with him. The old Indian from the previous cover has no connection with this special Master. On the cover of volume 2 the old Indian man is replaced by a drawing of me in meditation. It illustrates the fact that my spiritual journey after meeting Chariji is no longer focussed on India, but on the path to the innermost core of my heart. There is no longer any need to look outwards – for I have found my spiritual guide and Master ...

Happiness and the truth in life

During the moments when I am in touch with and feel the oneness with a high state and vibration, every desire for anything else than just being present in the now in this state disappears. I am convinced that "happiness" is not to be sought after in the external world, but that it is already – and has always been – at the innermost core of my heart.

When I am resting there, it is as if the external world does not exist. When I practice being in this inner state in my everyday life, and when I succeed, the state brings a deeper feeling of joy into everything I do.

The truth about life here on earth may be that in reality it is an illusion whose only purpose is to lead us humans to the next step towards the truth about life itself – the highest and eternal vibration.

Although I am not an expert, I have set my goal and charted my course. The spiritual path embraces the whole of my life in a positive way. With all my heart I wish to be a tool in the service of the highest. I will do my utmost to adjust and optimise this "tool" so that it can be of the greatest possible benefit.

In conclusion here is a quotation from one of the Vedic scriptures – from the Brihad-Aranyaka Upanishad – (see source 2 p. 127 verse 1.3.28). For me these three lines express the essence of the relationship between a student and his Master and to that which the Master can contribute:

*"From delusion lead me to Truth.
From darkness lead me to Light.
From death lead me to immortality."*

SOURCES

Sources concerning Indian spiritual philosophy and Hinduism

1) "I begyndelsen var der ingenting" article by Jens Gnaur, *Sahaj Marg Bladet* nr. 29
2) *The Upanishads* published by Penguin Classics with an introduction by Juan Mascaró
3) *The Rig Veda* published by Penguin Classics selected and translated by Wendy Doniger O'Flaherty
4) *Puranic Encyclopaedia* by Vettam Mani
5) Afsnittet: *Hymns of Rigveda and Atharvaveda Found in Yajurveda* on the website: http://www.hinduwebsite.com/sacredscripts/hinduism/yajur/Righymns.asp preface regarding Yajurveda written by R.T.H. Griffith
6) *Illustreret Religionshistorie* edited by Jes Peter Asmussen and Jørgen Læssøe
7) Gyldendal's encyclopedia *Den Store Danske* in the online edition, the article "Vedic religions" – see the following link: http://denstoredanske.dk/Sprog,_religion_og_filosofi/Religion_og_mystik/Indiske_religioner/vedareligion
8) *Om The Bhagavadgita or The Song Divine* by Gita Press, Gorakhpur, India
9) *Yoga, filosofi, asanas, pranayama* by Anne Lise Dresler
10) *Truth Eternal* by Shri Ram Chandraji (Lalaji)

11) *Liv Kommer Fra Liv* by Sri Srimad A.C. Bhaktivedanta Swami Prabhupada
12) *Ni upanishader* translated by Klara Preben-Hansen
13) *Politikens religionsleksikon* by Arild Hvidtfeldt
14) *Amrita Bindu Upanishad, from the Atharva Veda*, Translated by Swami Madhavanada, Published by Advaita Ashram, Kolkatta, see a pdf-version of the Amrita Bindu Upanishad on the website: http://www.arshabodha.org/shortupanishads/amritabinduupanishad.pdf
15) *Hindu Gods and Goddesses* by A.G. Mitchell
16) *The Symbolism of Hindu Gods and Rituals* by A. Parthasarathy
17) *Sadguru Dattatreya* by Sadguru Sant Keshavadas
18) *Taittereya Samhita* (Yajur) publ. by Harvard Oriental Series b. 18-19 translated by A.B Keith
19) *Atharva Veda* published by Harvard Oriental Series b. 7-8 translated by W.D. Whitney
20) *Atharvaveda* published by Sacred Books of the East b. 42 translated by M. Bloomfield
21) *Kaivalya Upanishad* – Translation with Notes: http://www.hinduwebsite.com/kaivalya.asp
22) *Lonely Planet Travel Survival Kit: India* published by Lonely Planet Publications
23) *Hinduismen* by Frede Møller-Kristensen
24) *Hindu Symbology and Other Essays* by Swami Swahananda
25) *The Mystery of Sri Chakra* by Sri Ganapati Sachchidananda Swamiji
26) *Jeg er Det* [the Danish version of: *I am that*] by Nisargadatta Maharaj

Sources concerning the four gurus

27) *The Mountain Path* by V. Ganesan published by Sri T.N. Venkataraman

Sources concerning the postscripts

28) *Yoga Sutras – How to know God* by Patañjali with commentary by Swami Prabhavananda and Christopher Isherwood (in the Danish version published by Visdomsbøgerne in 1983)
29) *Sahaj Marg Philosophy* by Ram Chandra (Babuji), part of the book: *Complete works of Ram Chandra, Volume I, 1th NAPCedition, 2nd reprint, 2009*
30) *Efficacy of Raja Yoga – in the light of Sahaj Marg* by Ram Chandra (Babuji), part of the book: *Complete works of Ram Chandra, Volume I, 1th NAPCedition, 2nd reprint, 2009*
31) *Reality at Dawn* by Ram Chandra (Babuji), part of the book: *Complete works of Ram Chandra, Volume I, 1th NAPCedition, 2nd reprint, 2009*
32) *Heart to Heart Volume IV, 2001* by P. Rajagopalachari (Chariji)
33) *Complete Works of Ram Chandra, Volume II, 1th NAPCedition, 2nd reprint, 2009* (Babuji)
34) *The Practice of Sahaj Marg – Role of the Abhyasi in Sahaj Marg* by P. Rajagopalachari (Chariji)
35) *Hvor Virkeligheden Begynder* by Ram Chandra (Babuji)
36) *What Is Sahaj Marg, 3rd edition 1995* by P. Rajagopalachari (Chariji)
37) *My Master – The Essence of Pure Love, 1995* by P. Rajagopalachari (Chariji)
38) *Love & Death, 1992* by P. Rajagopalachari (Chariji)

39) *Heart to Heart, Volume II, 1991* by P. Rajagopalachari (Chariji)
40) *Heart to Heart, Volume I, 1988* by P. Rajagopalachari (Chariji)
41) *Heart to Heart, Volume III, 1996* by P. Rajagopalachari (Chariji)
42) *The Practice of Sahaj Marg – Role of the Abhyasi in Sahaj Marg, 2009* by P. Rajagopalachari (Chariji)
43) *Combined Works of Chariji, Vol. 1, 2002* by P. Rajagopalachari (Chariji)
44) *HeartSpeak 2004, Volume II,* by P. Rajagopalachari (Chariji)
45) *The Yoga-Sūtras of Patañjali – Sanskrit English Translation & Glossary* by Chip Hartranft, 2003
46) *Patañjali's Yoga* with commentary by Vyâsa and glossary by Vâchaspati Mis'ra, 1974
47) *HeartSpeak 2005* by P. Rajagopalachari (Chariji)

Sources concerning some illustrations

I) The photo on the cover of this book was taken by photographer Sven Ulsa, Joy Postcards in India, who has kindly approved the use of it on the cover of both this volume one and the coming volume two – all rights reserved

II) The drawing page 9 in the book *The Symbolism of Hindu Gods and Rituals* (source 16), unknown artist, kindly lent by the author Mr. A. Parthasarathy at VedantaWorld in India, all rights reserved

III) The cover of the book *Sadguru Dattatreya* by Sadguru Sant Keshavadas (source 17), unknown artist, kindly lent by the author's son, Mr. Shyam Pai, all rights reserved

IV) The cover of the book *The Mystery of Sri Chakra* (source 25), unknown artist, kindly lent by Mr. Prasad, Swamiji's ashram, all rights reserved

V) Photo, unknown photographer, kindly lent by Mr. A. Sivasamy, all rights reserved
VI) Photo, unknown photographer, bought at Swamiji's ashram, unknown photographer, kindly lent by Swamiji, all rights reserved
VII) Photo, unknown photographer, bought at Sai Baba's ashram, kindly lent by Sri Sathya Sai Sadhana Trust, Publications Division, all rights reserved
VIII) Photo, unknown photographer, bought at Poonjaji's Satsang Bhavan, kindly lent by Sri Ramana Marhashi's Ashram, Sri Ramanasramam in India, all rights reserved
IX) Photo, unknown photographer, kindly lent by SRCM and Heartfulness Institute, all rights reserved
X) Photo, Eric Klitgaard, kindly lent by SRCM and Heartfulness Institute, all rights reserved
XI) Drawing, kindly lent by SRCM and Heartfulness Institute, all rights reserved

"Do what you have to do. Be divine in your essence. Be loving, be compassionate, be merciful. Treat everything as yourself…"

P. Rajagopalachari, Chariji, Heart to Heart Vol. V – page 232

"We each have our place in this universe, a unique place for every one of us. Never question the purpose for which you have been created. Try to find it. Try to fulfill it. That is what I believe is the final message of Sahaj Marg."

P. Rajagopalachari, Chariji, HeartSpeak 2004 Vol. I – page 58

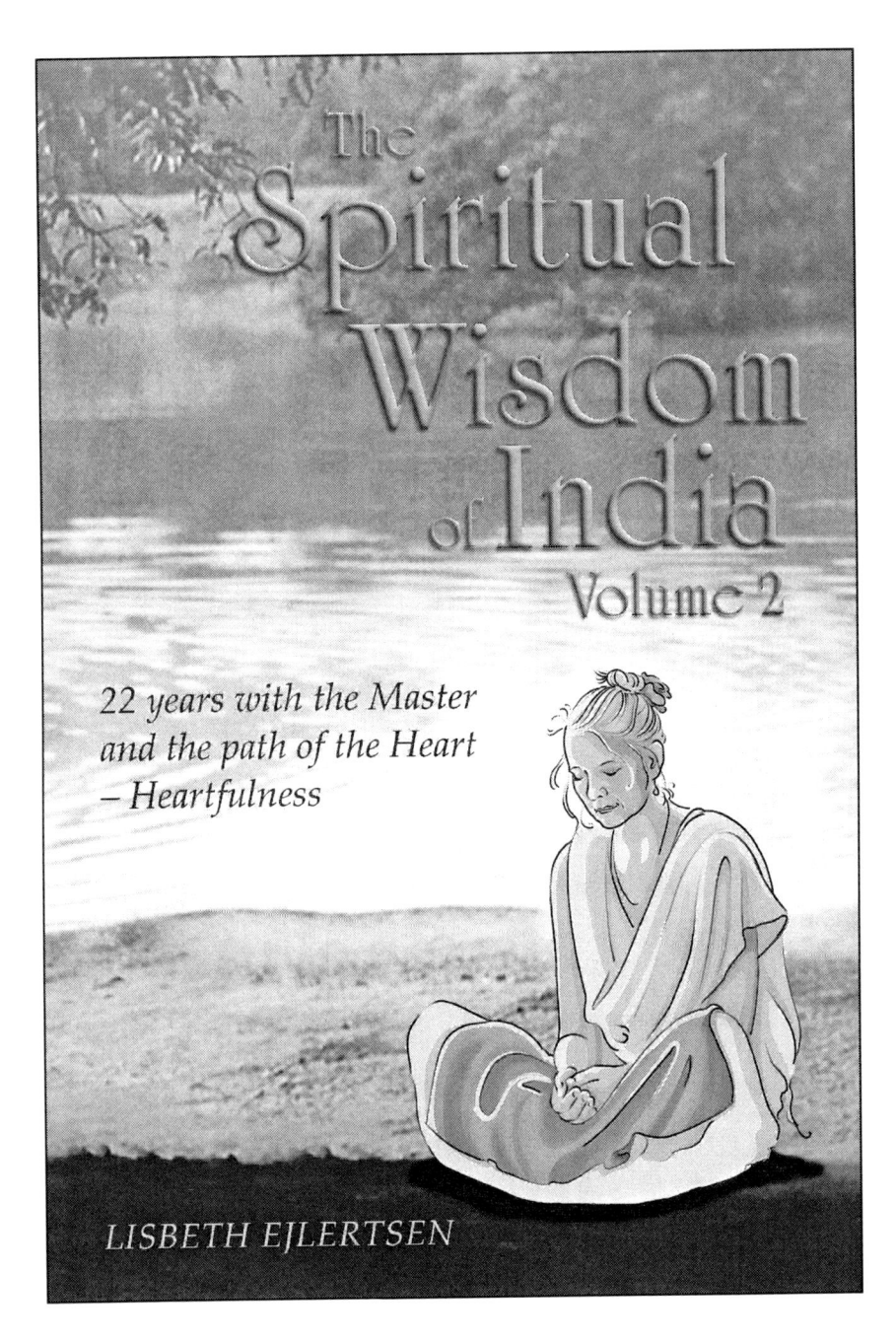

The Spiritual Wisdom of India
Volume 2

22 years with the Master and the path of the Heart – Heartfulness

LISBETH EJLERTSEN

The cover of the next volume of this book:
"The Spiritual Wisdom of India, Volume 2" with the subtitle:
"22 years with the Master and the path of the Heart – Heartfulness"

VOLUME 2 – WILL BE PUBLISHED IN AUTUMN 2017

A true Master is with you in your heart ...

- Why follow a spiritual Master?
- How do you achieve confidence in a Master?
- What benefits can be gained from a Master?

Lisbeth Ejlertsen grew up in the culture of the West. In spite of her Danish roots, she chose to follow a Master of Indian origin in 1995. She followed her heart's desire ...

You will gain insight into Lisbeth's past 22 years with the Master – and learn how a Master can touch a heart and the experiences which step by step caused Lisbeth to open up for a closer inner contact with her Master.

You will gain inspiration through her personal deliberations and experiences which bear witness to both good and bad times, to easy and difficult steps, to valuable and inexplicable experiences and about choosing to flow with life.

Lisbeth's experiences show how reality can be changed in the split second that you adjust your own inner perspective.

What is your heart's desire?

If you would like to read more about volume 2 – please visit:

www.thespiritualwisdomofindia.com

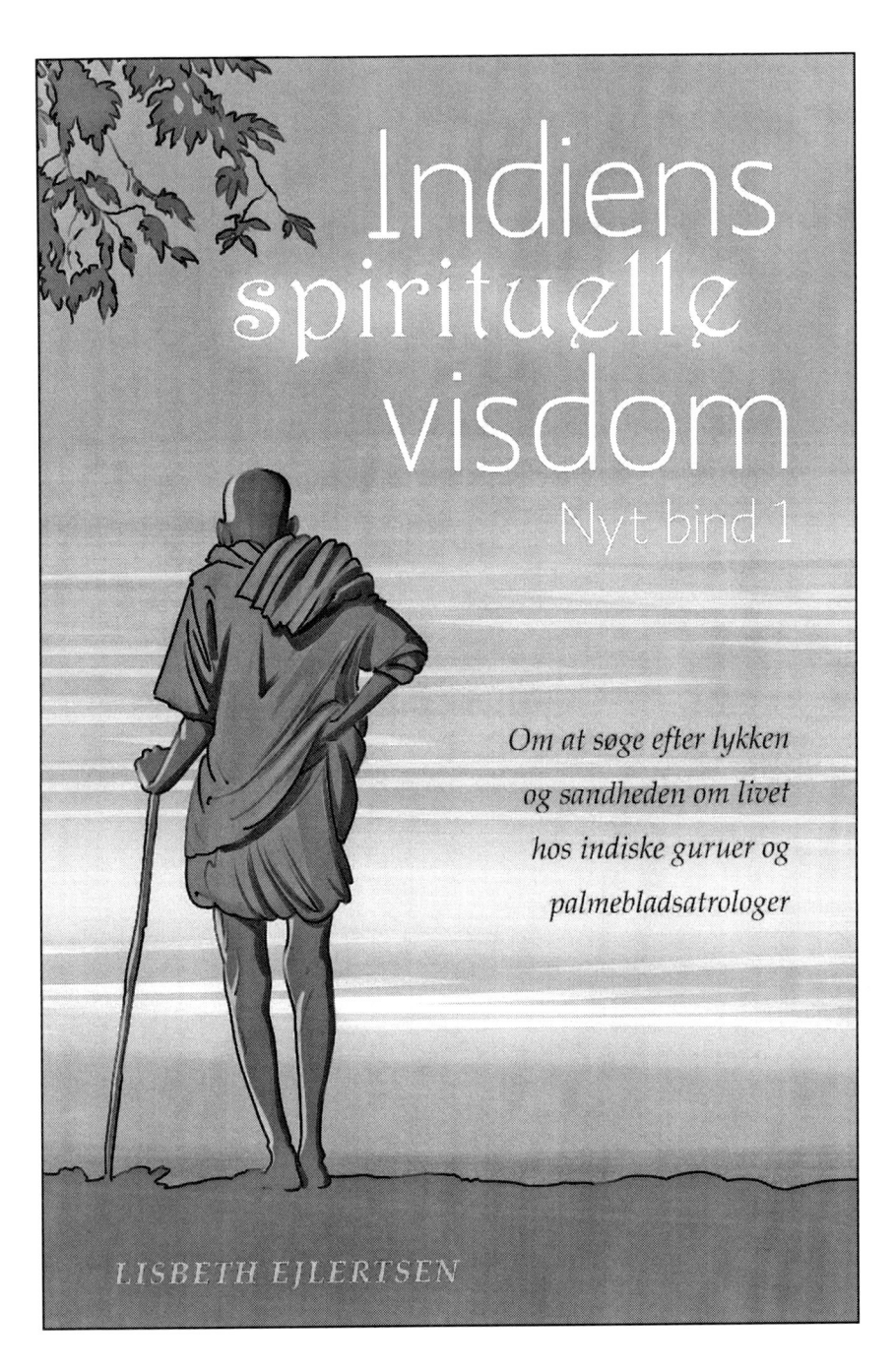

The cover of the Danish volume of this book. Photo: Lent by FlowLab

THIS BOOK – ALSO IN DANISH

The Danish edition of this book has the following Danish title and subtitle:

Indiens spirituelle visdom, Nyt bind 1

Om at søge efter lykken og sandheden om livet
hos indiske guruer og palmebladsastrologer

If you like to read more about the Danish book – in Danish – please use:

www.indiensspirituellevisdom.dk

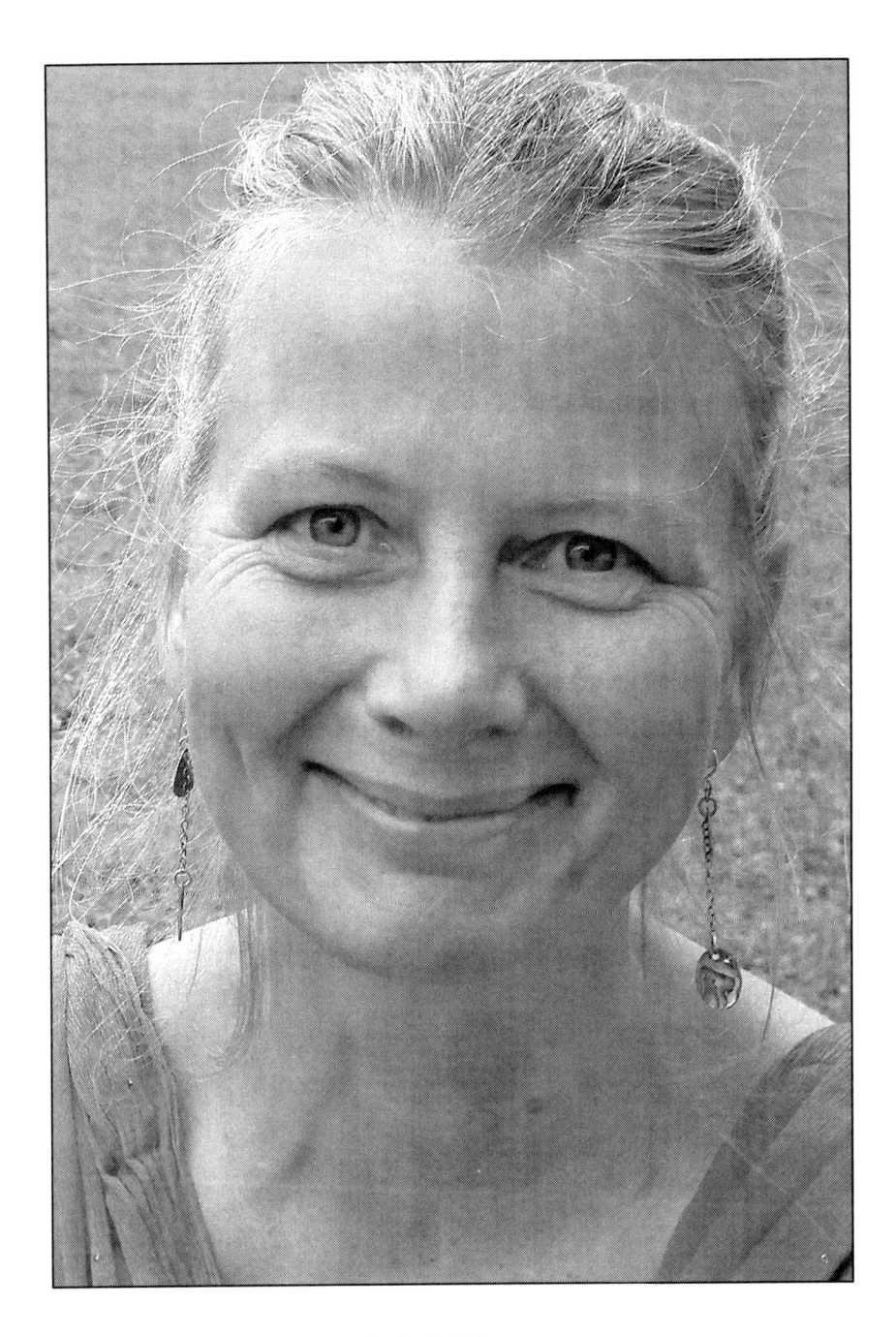

Lisbeth Ejlertsen
Foto: Gunver Mossin Kofoed

ABOUT THE AUTHOR

Throughout her whole life Lisbeth Ejlertsen has been fascinated with inner life and what makes us happy. Her life's work has been to explore the human capacities that lie within each of us and to make those potentials visible to others.

For most of her adult life Lisbeth has listened to and followed her inner voice. This has led her to meditate for at least 30 years, follow a spiritual master for more than 20 years and visit India more than 20 times in order to explore the richness of the spiritual wisdom this country offers.

In 1991, she chose to say goodbye to a career in engineering and to follow her inner call to start a business where she could focus on developing and arranging courses about "Flow" in life. She also began writing, painting and working as a trauma therapist.

These days Lisbeth lives in Vrads, a small village surrounded by beautiful Danish countryside and close to the meditation center where she continues to absorb herself in the infinite paths of development of the heart.

If you like to read more – please use:

www.lisbethejlertsen.com

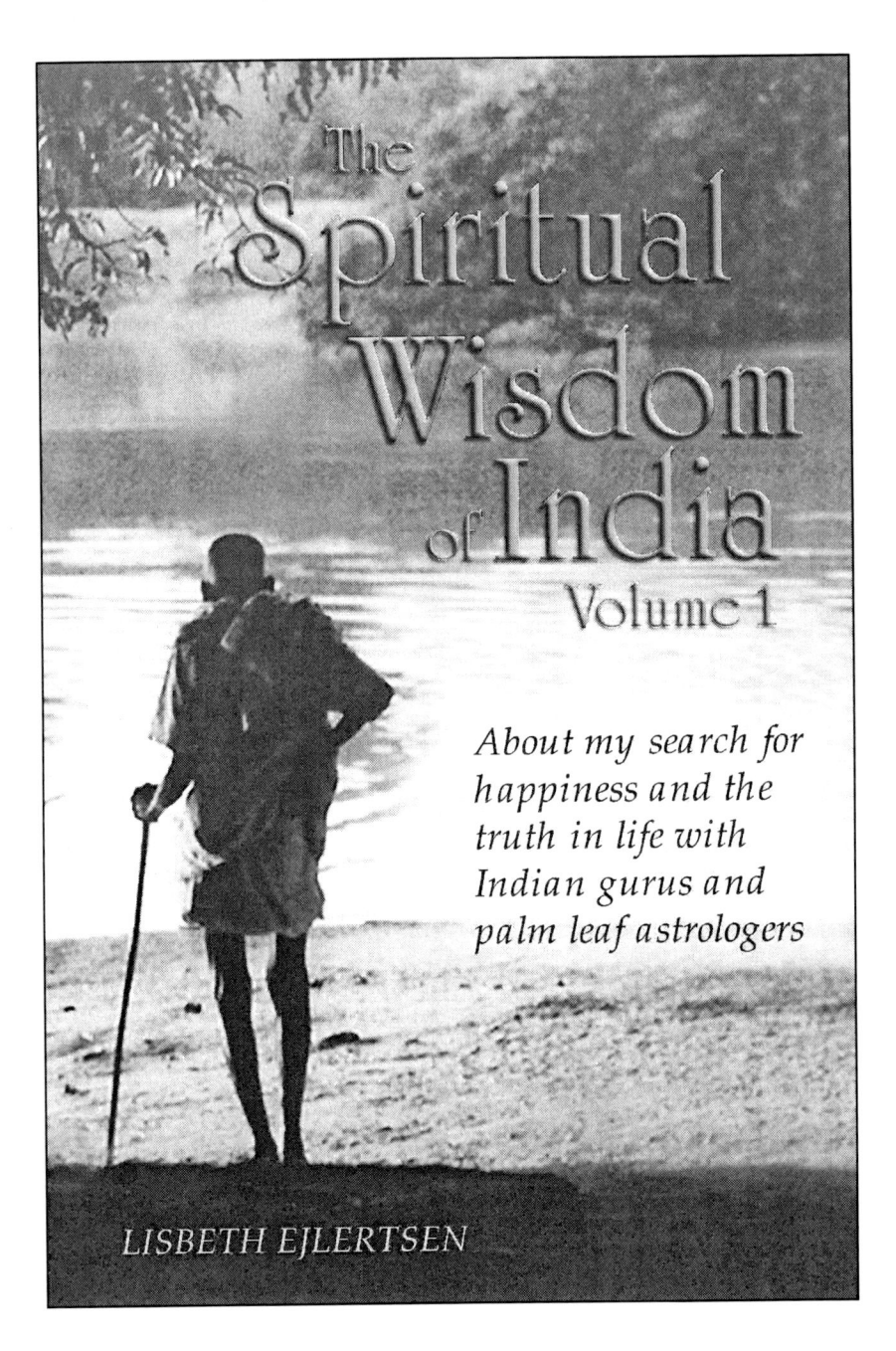

The cover of this book: "The Spiritual Wisdom of India, Volume 1" with the subtitle: "About my search for happiness and the truth in life with Indian gurus and palm leaf astrologers"

THIS BOOK – VOLUME 1

Where do you find happiness and the truth in life?

In 1994, curiosity and the urge for adventure brought Lisbeth Ejlertsen to India where she carried these questions in her heart:

- Does life have a purpose?
- Is there a way to eternal happiness?
- Is our fate predestined?

She wanted to search for the answer to the mystery of life with spiritual teachers and palm leaf astrologers in the country that has given pride of place to spirituality for centuries.

It is said of the gurus that they have access to special levels in the universe, and the centuries' old palm leaf archives are believed to hold predictions about the life courses of human beings. Could the mystery of life and Lisbeth's destiny be written in higher realms or on approximately 2000 year old palm leaves …?

You will gain insight into the wisdom of the oldest scriptures in the world, the Vedas, into spiritual concepts and into Lisbeth's surprising and overwhelming experiences, which a Western approach to life cannot explain.

On her spiritual course up until 2017, you will meet Heartfulness – a unique way of accessing the heart which unites people and helps each individual to find inner tranquillity and balance.

Would you like to go with her out into world and into the heart?

If you would like to read more about this book – please visit:

www.thespiritualwisdomofindia.com

REVIEWS

You can read the reviews of both the English and the Danish edition of the book on the website for the book. Please follow this link:

www.thespiritualwisdomofindia.com/reviews/

The professional American book reviewer, The US Review of Books, wrote among other things the following:

The Spiritual Wisdom of India by Lisbeth Ejlertsen, AuthorHouse
Reviewed by Jennifer Hummer

"The five gurus who I met on my way all had the same message; that happiness is to be united with the divine in oneself; everything is in being."

… The author does a good job simplifying Eastern topics such as Sanskrit, Mantra, Vedas and the Bhagavadgita (the Hindu "Bible") to name just a few. Her easy and unintimidating writing style allows both novices and experts alike to absorb her stories and teachings without feeling naïve or judged. With her extended wealth of information on the spiritual wisdom of India, Ejlersten might just be called a master herself.

RECOMMENDED by the US Review

©2017 All Rights Reserved • The US Review of Books